THE GIFTS OF WINTER

Dr Stephanie Fitzgerald is a chartered clinical psychologist, neuropsychologist, and Associate Fellow of the British Psychological Society. She is also a keynote speaker and the author of four previous books, including *Reworked: Putting health and happiness at the centre of your career*, and workbooks on anxiety and OCD.

She has worked in mental health for two decades, including ten years for the NHS, before moving to private practice to coach individuals who feel burned out, overwhelmed, stressed and anxious. She also provides professional wellbeing support to companies across varying industries, including rail, aerospace, civil engineering and Premier League football.

THE GIFTS OF WINTER

How to uncover seasonal joy, health and happiness

DR STEPHANIE FITZGERALD

MICHAEL JOSEPH

PENGUIN MICHAEL JOSEPH

UK | USA | Canada | Ireland | Australia
India | New Zealand | South Africa

Penguin Michael Joseph is part of the Penguin Random House group of companies whose addresses can be found at global.penguinrandomhouse.com

Penguin Random House UK,
One Embassy Gardens, 8 Viaduct Gardens, London SW11 7BW

penguin.co.uk

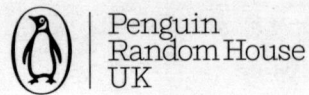

First published 2025

001

Copyright © Dr Stephanie Fitzgerald, 2025
Internal illustrations copyright © Ryn Frank, 2025

The moral right of the author has been asserted

This book is a work of non-fiction based on the life, experiences and recollections of the author. In some cases names of people, places, dates, sequences and the detail of events have been changed to protect the privacy of others

The information in this book is intended for general guidance only. Whilst every effort has been made to ensure that the information is complete and accurate, it is not a substitute for medical or healthcare professional advice. Please consult with your GP or a qualified health professional before changing, stopping or starting any treatment or medication. All matters regarding your health require medical supervision. The author and publishers disclaim, as far as the law allows, any liability arising directly or indirectly from the use, or misuse, of the information in this book

No part of this book may be used or reproduced in any manner for the purpose of training artificial intelligence technologies or systems. In accordance with Article 4(3) of the DSM Directive 2019/790, Penguin Random House expressly reserves this work from the text and data mining exception

Set in 14/17.7pt Bembo Book MT Pro
Typeset by Six Red Marbles UK, Thetford, Norfolk
Printed and bound in Great Britain by Clays Ltd, Elcograf S.p.A.

The authorized representative in the EEA is Penguin Random House Ireland, Morrison Chambers, 32 Nassau Street, Dublin D02 YH68

A CIP catalogue record for this book is available from the British Library

ISBN: 978–0–241–77957–6

Penguin Random House is committed to a sustainable future for our business, our readers and our planet. This book is made from Forest Stewardship Council® certified paper

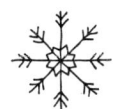

*For my beautiful sister Laura,
to help you embrace winter's hug x*

Contents

Introduction ... 1

Chapter 1: Making space for winter ... 5
Chapter 2: A winter mood ... 19
Chapter 3: A shift in mindset ... 30
Chapter 4: Embracing a winter break ... 44
Chapter 5: A winter retreat at home ... 54
Chapter 6: A winter bedtime ... 68
Chapter 7: The fabric of winter ... 89
Chapter 8: The taste of winter ... 104
Chapter 9: Winter's light ... 125
Chapter 10: Getting out in winter ... 135
Chapter 11: Moving through winter ... 150
Chapter 12: Learning to love and celebrate in winter ... 164
Chapter 13: A calm(er) Christmas ... 178
Chapter 14: A winter garden ... 202
Chapter 15: The practical preparations for winter ... 216
Chapter 16: A beginning, a middle and an end ... 229

Epilogue: The words of winter ... 247
Acknowledgements ... 255
Endnotes ... 257
Index ... 269
Notes ... 277

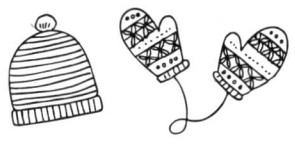

Introduction

There are gifts in winter. Threads of magic woven through the fabric of the season. They lie in the whispered words of nature, inviting us to settle into the hush. Winter is a time of recovery and preparation, offering us the chance for cosy contentedness and so much more. There is a sparkle of wonder, a peppiness and a vitality that has the power to restore and revive us.

Although winter arrives much more quietly than other seasons, slipping in under the darkest shadows of autumn, it brings with it unexpected lightness and vibrancy. Its charms may appear hidden in the depths of the cold and the dark but, just beneath the surface, there lies beauty, joy and contentment, waiting to be found.

There is much to cherish in winter, but it's easy to lose sight of this. With the everyday rush of life and global events leaving us tired and diminished, winter can feel like one extra challenge we could do without. The story we are told is wholly negative. We are sold a season of nothingness. A fallow and barren period. The rhetoric from every angle is how awful and miserable it is, something to be endured. No wonder we try to shut winter out, drawing the curtains against the darkness. If we go into any situation thinking, 'I can't stand this, I want it to be over,' then our experiences will almost certainly align with that way of thinking. We cannot experience the delight and awe of winter if we keep our heads down, avoiding and wishing it away.

It may seem surprising that I now love winter. Whilst I was always upbeat about the season throughout my childhood and early twenties, after suffering several years of crippling seasonal affective disorder (SAD), together with some challenging personal events which occurred at this time of year, I was left feeling despondent and overwhelmed. My dread of winter cloaked me in heavy negativity, not just throughout winter itself but also pre-emptively, starting with the very thought of the season approaching.

Back then, I did everything I could to ignore and reject winter, overcommitting at work and cramming my schedule so full that I'd barely have time to breathe, let alone acknowledge the season around me. I was exhausted but hoped that I could distract myself away from winter. I kept my head down and waited for it to be over but, even from the depths of my dislike, I knew there was a better way. I've been a psychologist for over two decades, specializing in neuropsychology for nearly 15 years. I'm fascinated by how our brains interact with our surroundings. In recent years, I have watched our attitudes towards winter become more and more negatively skewed and knew it wasn't working for us. The way I myself approached winter every year not only bruised my heart but was actively going against my professional knowledge, and it wasn't serving me well. I felt in my gut that winter had more to offer me and that, somehow, its gifts had become buried under my own experiences and challenges. I realized that it wasn't winter itself that I hated and wanted to avoid, but how I *felt* in winter. It wasn't winter; it was me. I knew from my clinical practice that I wasn't alone.

I needed to do something about it. I needed solutions. I wanted the understanding, the tools and the capability to better manage my mental and physical health during a season when the odds felt fully stacked against me. And I didn't want to fake it. As Welsh author Horatio Clare writes in his book *The Light in the Dark*: 'It does not do to romanticize drizzle, rain on motorways, months of strip lighting, office windows black at four o'clock and concrete skies.'[1] I knew I couldn't simply *will* myself to start liking winter again, and as an evidence-based practitioner, I wanted more. I began an exploration, seeking the science and practical advice I needed in order to do winter better.

On my voyage of discovery, I developed so much more than a survival guide; I fell deeply in love with winter. I discovered a magic that I never knew existed. Once I started seeking the beauty of the season, I couldn't escape it. Every day, I found something new, and these experiences embedded themselves as pockets of joy in my heart.

Winter is a captivating and truly gorgeous season, but too often we refuse to engage with it. We block it out. Winter offers us a restorative period of rest and reflection, an antidote to the chaos of the year, but we rush past with our summer energy and unchanging routines. By ignoring the spectacular beauty of winter, we miss out on an opportunity that no other season presents.

That's why I wrote this book. I want to encourage everyone not to romanticize winter, but to truly lean into winter's embrace. Winter hasn't abandoned us, and we shouldn't abandon winter. Consider this book your treasure map, revealing where the hidden gems of winter are and what you can do to find them. It normalizes why and when the season is tough and shares practical tips for overcoming the challenges. You will no longer be gritting your teeth to get through it. Instead, you will be held through winter, by winter. You'll feel support, solace and succour.

This book will guide you through the challenges and what we can do to overcome them but also introduce you to the magic we so often overlook. With easy-to-implement tips alongside regular points of reflection throughout, you will begin to break down the blockers that stop you from engaging with the season and learn how your body and brain can thrive at this time of year. You will uncover and engage with the warmth, joy, health and happiness woven into winter.

We all experience the challenges of home, health, work and family that tumble around in the kaleidoscope of life throughout the year. But one thing we needn't do is *battle* winter. Since discovering another way to approach the season, I have felt happiness and contentment. My soul has been settled. I've experienced joy, encouragement, playful energy and a full heart, all of which are gifts from winter. Now I want you to experience them too.

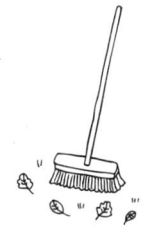

Chapter 1: Making space for winter

Do you make space for winter? Take a moment to consider. Do you put time and energy into making seasonal adjustments? What changes in your world in winter? If your answer is 'nothing', then you are not alone. Many of us head into the season without giving it any thought, only paying attention when we realize that we are finding it hard. There is no doubt that winter itself can pose some challenges, but it is not fully responsible for the obstacles we face. These are not the direct result of winter but rather challenges that we create ourselves.

One such challenge is our absolute refusal to make adjustments. There is a direct link between how much space we create for winter and how comfortable we will find the season. I see time and again that we refuse to make a single adaptation to the season, continuing with the same activities, pace and diet of summer, and then we state that winter is hard. Yet winter doesn't have to make life hard. Quite the opposite.

Winter is full of invitations. *Stop. Rest. Put down your tools.*

Look, I'll turn down the lights for you. How do we respond? By flicking on the electric lights. Winter gently encourages us to prioritize ourselves: *Why don't you have some sensory rest so you feel refreshed and restored?* What do we do? We swipe our way through the lives of thousands of strangers online, absorbing views, information and opinions far faster than we can ever hope to process. We drown in a sea of stimulation in a moment where winter invites us to sit quietly and savour the hush. Winter cools the air around us, encouraging us to go to bed, to snuggle, to tell stories and to connect. We, in turn, crank up the heating and sit far apart on the sofa, scrolling small screens in front of big screens. Our modern world shouts loudly and brashly over the softly spoken words of winter, which, if we listen, invite us to sit and *be*, together. The truth is that we make our own lives harder and then blame our challenges on winter.

We are no longer aligned with when nature's heartbeat quickens and slows. There is a natural ebb and flow to the year's energy, but we choose to ignore it. Instead, we try to maintain a steady pace throughout the year and then wonder why we are so exhausted at the end of it. We make zero adjustments, then blame winter for our depleted energy.

It's 5.45am on a mid-January morning and I am scraping ice off my car windscreen in the dark. I am heading to the gym, which is only down the road and opens at 6am. Why am I shivering in an inadequate hoodie at this ridiculous hour, trying to clear my car and getting ready to drive? Because that's what I do. That's my routine. Or rather, that was my routine. All through the summer, I (almost) enjoyed getting up at 5.30am, having a quick cup of tea and hopping in the car at 5.55am, ready to swipe my membership card and be in position to kickstart both my workout and my day by 6.01am.

So, what's wrong with this picture? Well, I'm not hopping in my car at 5.55am. I am instead having to allow an additional 10 minutes or so to clear the car windscreen, leaving the engine running and praying that my neighbours don't hate me too much for it (spoiler alert: they do). I'm not enjoying a cup of tea before I head out; I'm making it in a to-go cup to have en route and I feel weird taking a sip of tea instead of the more conventional glug of water on the treadmill. What's wrong with this picture is that I haven't made any space for winter.

All through summer, I loved the sense of achievement that came from knowing I was ahead of the crowd by getting my workout done. I felt a sense of smugness in the near-empty gym and felt more dedicated than those who chose to stay in bed. But that smugness fades now as I realize I'm literally running on empty. I don't have any energy, but I am feeling extra pressure to make my workout worthwhile, as it took so much more effort to get here. I think about my friends who turned off their early alarms and committed to more sleep and can't help but question if I really am living the healthier lifestyle after all.

I am not alone. Very few of us change our lifestyles with the seasons because, thanks to modern living, we don't have to. Everything from electricity to international shipping means our patterns, routines, rhythms and diet are no longer dictated by daylight hours or temperature. We can ignore the seasons as we push on through with our own routines and plans, but nature, as always, is more powerful than us. Its impact is felt whether we choose to pay attention to it or not.

You may well say to me, 'It's not my fault, my life doesn't allow for adjustments or changes.' But that's not winter's fault either. We cannot blame winter for not matching our summer-energy lifestyle. We create disappointment in one season when we carry over the expectations of another. It is as though we wish for the sun but grumble when presented with the moon. Both are magical, mystical, full of promise and purpose, but we are guaranteed to miss the beauty and healing strength of the moon if we spend the entire time looking around it for the sun.

Before we can experience a better winter, we have to acknowledge the part *we* play in making winter difficult. Yes, winter poses some challenges, but so does every season. Even summer, which 42% of us cite as our favourite season,[1] requires us to overlook the hay fever, the sweaty discomfort at night, and the moments of relentless heat keeping us in what Jane Austen described as 'a continual state of inelegance'.[2]

We don't gain anything from trying to squeeze winter out of our year and pretend it's not happening. We don't need to learn how to 'survive' winter because, in fact, winter comes laden with gifts. If we listen, winter might say to us, *Look, I know this can be tough. I'm going to bring a little more light every day. I'm going to bring peace, gentleness, a sense of calm and clarity. I am going to offer you a chance to slow down, and I will hold you tightly and safely until you are ready to greet the world again.*

Winter offers us everything we need; we just have to budge up and make space for it. We cannot find the good in winter without truly engaging with it. The rewards we get will rejuvenate us for the rest of the year and the higher-energy seasons ahead. Making space for winter means making small adjustments to welcome the season and the energetic shift that it brings. It is minimal effort for maximum reward. It is so worth investing this time to overcome the challenges and gain the benefits from the most restorative season of the year.

The never-ending winter

When it comes to challenges, one element of winter definitely occupies more than its fair share of the season. Whether you celebrate it or not, it is the reason why winter can feel never-ending and explains why so often we are ready for winter to be over before it has even really begun. That element is, of course, Christmas.

In the UK, Christmas begins to creep onto our shelves and into our consciousness from September onwards. September. As in summer-has-just-left-the-building September. We are being sold Christmas before autumn has barely made an appearance, let alone winter. We are forced to think about Christmas a good four months ahead of the event itself. None of this early hard sell is designed to help us. We may be sold ideas of planning ahead and spreading the cost, but as many an outraged headline has pointed out, much Christmas food is sold with a use-by date that pre-dates the big day itself.

Early Christmas stock is not brought into stores for our benefit. Magazines that want to publish a 'best Christmas display' or 'where to buy the best mince pie' feature are working to submit their December issue for publication in October. This means the shops need to be prepared, Christmas goodies must be displayed, lights must be switched on, etc. in plenty of time for journalists to examine it all. Then articles are written and opinions are shared, which will influence what we do, or don't, buy to celebrate Christmas.

And so it begins. In September. We browse beneath twinkling fairy lights. We shop to Christmas number one hits, pushing our trolleys around humming, 'Simply . . . having . . . a wonderful Christmas time,' and who hasn't given it their all along with Mariah when she first plays through our car stereos? We play the game, we join in, we're involved . . . and then we're fed up. No wonder! What other event in the year has a four-month build-up? When else would we ask people to maintain a level of enthusiasm and excitement for so long, other than perhaps a wedding? (Even then, at some point, the happy couple have likely exchanged a glance over table plans that translates to 'we should have eloped'.)

With such a long build-up to Christmas, many people are completely fed up with 'winter' before it has technically begun. By Boxing Day, we've had enough and are ready for spring, even though winter has barely been with us for 72 hours. Even if you don't celebrate Christmas or you celebrate another religious or secular event around this time, unless you stay at home from September to December, you cannot avoid the chaos. We are inundated with Christmas commercialism, and it leaves us physically, mentally and financially exhausted.

Later on, we'll explore how to have a better Christmas/holiday season, so I won't dwell on this too much here other than to say that if Christmas really dominates and drains your winter of joy and energy, or if it leaves you feeling emotionally depleted, then fear not. Winter also offers a wonderful antidote to all the Christmas noise and chaos that we face, with nearly three months of potential restoration and re-energizing to take advantage of. If we want to experience the season differently, then we need to break away from the commercial calendar and reframe our year. There is a different way to approach winter, a way that could make us much happier. Only it might not be what you think.

Rewriting your year

There are many ways to define a season. Astronomical seasons refer to the position of the earth's orbit in relation to the sun.[3] It is the astronomical seasons that are responsible for the spring equinox when the clocks go forward and the autumn equinox when the clocks go back (my personal favourite: hello, extra hour in bed!). This definition of the seasons sees winter start around 20 December and spring start around 20 March.

Then we have the meteorological seasons, which consist of splitting the seasons into four three-month periods, coinciding with our Gregorian calendar. This sees the seasons divided into winter as December/January/February, spring as March/April/May, summer as June/July/August and autumn as September/October/November.

So far, so inconsistent. One definition has winter starting at the beginning of December; the other has winter starting three weeks later. Then the workplace can complicate matters further by dividing our year into quarters, with 'Q1' starting in January. This corporate calendar adds a layer of complexity and a further blocker to us tuning into the seasons around us. We set ourselves up to begin afresh in Q1, to push projects with renewed energy and vigour and to start new initiatives just as we enter into the restorative slow-down phase of nature.

This is why, in a sentence I never thought I would utter, I believe the tax year could make us happier. Let me explain.

The UK tax year sees the start of the year begin from 1 April. We're in good company, with Japan, Canada, Hong Kong, Singapore and South Africa all running their fiscal years from 1 April to 31 March.[4] I am suggesting that we do the same: not just with our finances but with our personal approach to the year. The calendar year and the traditions we follow don't allow us to *celebrate* winter. Instead, we give it a week to ten days maximum, and then we want rid of it. Could we let ourselves embrace winter if we rewrote the layout of our year?

Imagine seeing April as the start of the new year, where you initiate goals and plans using the energy of the awakening spring. All the build-up, expectation and hope you pour into a new year would have an extra three months from January to March to burgeon. Wouldn't that feel less exhausting? Wouldn't that allow you to plan, restore, accommodate and settle into winter more in the meantime? The thing is, we *can*. It's as simple as rewriting our year. The reason the way we currently do things feels wrong is because we are fighting against nature. Timing our new year goals with the beginning of spring would tune us into the rhythm of the seasons, making an enormous difference to us, our energy and the rest of the year. It's a simple change, but it's powerful.

Activity: Rewrite your year

Rewrite your year right now by dividing it into April–June (spring), July–September (summer), October–December (autumn), January–March (winter). Now mark 1 April as New Year's Day. This shift in mindset allows for a very different winter. You now have January to March to plan, plot and recharge, ready for the year ahead. You can now align your energy with the seasons.

You can embrace the crisp, glittering January mornings, the slow thaw of the garden, the gentle budding of trees and the hailing rain of March, knowing that it is *supposed* to be that way. Spring would feel so much more authentic if we began it with gentle April showers leading into (hopefully) months of glorious sunshine.

> This rewrite of the year better aligns with our energies, our seasons, our weather, our . . . everything. This way, winter becomes a period to look forward to. To enjoy, not endure. We can sink into three extra months of cosy bliss, relieving the pressure to get up and get going until we have gathered the energy and the resources to do so. Doesn't that sound positive? Doesn't that sound better?
>
> I began to rewrite my calendar a couple of years ago, and now I really look forward to winter. It has become my recharging station of the year, and I feel the earth's energy shift with me, supporting my year ahead. It's a glorious approach and really could make you happier, just as it has done for me. Can you make the shift right now to mentally start your new year on 1 April? How does it make you feel knowing that you've bought yourself three more months before it's all systems go? I know I feel lighter and more positive as the tension eases from my shoulders. Who would have believed that the tax year could make you happier?

Screeching to a halt

The opposite of budging up and making space for winter is a complete stopping. Not so much an adjustment as a checking out of the season altogether.

My partner and I are sitting in a café with my friend Claire and her husband, Jacob. We're having the type of slightly strained catch-up that comes with two bored children being forced to sit with two childless grown-ups who like kids but are not experienced enough to entertain them.

Jacob is on particularly bad form, snapping at the kids and overreacting when his smallest tries to clamber onto his knee, knocking his phone out of his hand in the process. I gently ask him what's wrong. He gruffly says 'nothing' before admitting that he's feeling out of sorts, a bit depressed and a bit agitated. He says he doesn't want to talk about it. Seeking safe ground, I ask him how his running is going, and he says, 'I've stopped for winter now.' I hesitate. My inner psychologist is desperate, positively *itching*, to point out that of course he's struggling. Jacob is a runner. A proper runner. None of this wheezing along, glancing at your watch and wondering if 0.3 miles can be rounded up to the 5km that was your original intention when you set out (just me?). Jacob runs four times a week, casually cracking out 10 to 15 miles at a time. He often gets up at 5am to squeeze some miles in before work. Jacob is a runner. Only now, he isn't. Now it is cold and dark, he has decided that running isn't for him, so now he's not doing anything.

I gently ask him if he thinks this could be affecting his mood. If having relied on regular doses of endorphins and oxytocin, all feel-good and repairing hormones, his brain might be wondering where all the good stuff has gone. What is he doing to stress-bust now? Jacob's answer: 'Nothing.' He hasn't adapted his routine; he's ground to a halt.

You don't need to be a psychologist to see how problematic this is. Jacob's belief that running and winter do not go together means he stopped completely but then struggled emotionally. This is a classic example of how we blame winter for ruining things when, in reality, the rigidity in Jacob's approach to exercise is the problem. Jacob needed to recognize that a reasonable adjustment had to be made. His routine needed to look a little different to accommodate the changes that naturally come with winter. He didn't need to stop. He needed to make space for winter. When he didn't, he struggled.

Making reasonable adjustments

The first step to making space for winter is working out *what* we need to make space for. Sometimes, we have a carefully curated plan or set of objectives for the year, but life has other ideas and we are thrown off course. This is why it's important to regularly tune into your feelings, energy and expectations throughout the year, and especially in the run-up to winter.

Try to let go of any assumptions you have about yourself. I've found that blanket beliefs such as 'I'm a morning person' shift and change during different seasons. Instead, we can uncover what we are *actually* feeling and what we might need to make space for.

🔋 Activity: Make an energy timeline

Take a blank piece of paper, or grab your journal, and draw a timeline of your previous year, from 12 months ago to the present month. This doesn't need to be beautiful, just a simple line with 12 marks along it denoting the months of the year. Now plot your energy according to how you felt throughout the year. Which were your high-energy months and when did you chill out? Has your year held regular breaks and moments for restoration or has it been a steady uphill climb with no reprieve? Have you had chaotic months?

Whatever the energetic timeline of your year looks like, don't judge it. This isn't a time for harsh words or recrimination. It's a time for noticing. When we see how our year has been to date, we can see what has worked well for us and what we may need now. This, in turn, tells us what we need to make space for.

If you notice that your winter held many expectations, plans and high-energy New Year's resolutions, or if your year has felt like one continual effort with little reprieve, I encourage you to do this next year differently and implement the changes that will make winter into your safe space. A space where you can regroup. Where you can gather together your thoughts, your plans and your joy. Winter can become your place of peace, offering rest.

A place to be in harmony with nature. It is the one time of year when you can deeply exhale and let go of high-energy pressure, not least from yourself.

There is a big difference between stagnancy and stillness, and this is not a stagnant season. Much is going on beneath the surface. Winter is our charging pad, awaiting us like a warm hug that we can walk into to refuel and replenish for the year ahead. What do you need from winter this year? What will you make space for?

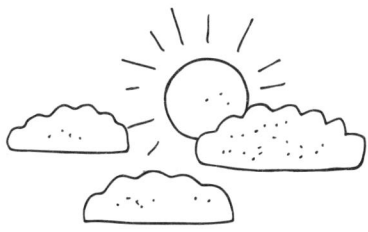

Chapter 2:
A winter mood

On telling people I was writing a book about winter, I was often asked, 'Is it about seasonal affective disorder?' This book is not aimed exclusively at those who have SAD. After all, we *all* go through winter every year, with or without SAD. However, I couldn't write about winter mood without acknowledging the challenges that SAD presents. If you've never heard of SAD, it is a type of depression that comes and goes in a seasonal pattern. It is most commonly seen in winter, when symptoms are more apparent and severe, although some people may experience SAD in summer.

I want to share my own experiences of SAD because it presented me with two sides of the winter coin. On the one hand, having SAD prevented me from seeing the gifts of winter. I wrote off the entire season and would feel panicky from the summer solstice onwards, a sense of dread settling in my stomach and weighing on my heart once I knew darker days were coming. On the other hand, in seeking ways to better manage my SAD, I discovered a whole world of brightness, care and support, and my eyes were opened to a winter that I never knew existed. I would never say I am thankful for my SAD because it would be disingenuous to pretend that I'm ever grateful for any episode of depression, but I am grateful for what it taught me. What it showed me. What it prompted in me. I am grateful for what I discovered and grateful that I can share that with you in this book.

Winter is such a comforting and compassionate season in so many ways, but we have to recognize our mood in order to embrace the opportunity for self-care that winter affords us. It is very natural and normal to experience a slump in mood over winter. We'll come on to look at the difference between winter blues and SAD and how to best manage your winter mood. But I want to start with SAD because, for me, learning about it was a game changer.

SAD can be dismissed as feeling low or lethargic over winter, but the symptoms mirror those seen in depression and wider depressive disorders. I won't dwell too much on symptoms here, not least because it's too easy to see familiar symptoms and rush to diagnose ourselves. However, I do want to emphasize the mirroring of symptoms of depression because the impacts can be severe. Those impacted by SAD may experience a persistent low mood, regardless of current life events. Often individuals may cry without being able to identify a cause or express why they feel unhappy. They may experience a loss of interest in hobbies or pleasurable activities. As a consequence, they may withdraw and no longer participate in activities or social events, which, in turn, increases feelings of isolation and depression. Cravings for carbohydrates are common because the brain seeks additional serotonin, which can be synthesized in response to carbs. In this way, it is not uncommon for individuals to self-medicate with high-carbohydrate foods in an attempt to boost their mood. There can be impacts on memory, concentration and sleep. Some individuals may experience hypersomnia, where they spend many extra hours sleeping, or indeed struggle to get out of bed at all. Others will battle with insomnia. Unfortunately, it is not uncommon for people with SAD to experience suicidal thoughts, which can be exceptionally scary for both the individuals and those around them.

I mentioned that we have a tendency to self-diagnose when we see a list of symptoms, and depression is no different. Our mood operates on a spectrum, and we may recognize some of these symptoms as those that we experience every now and then, or in response to life events. The above does not represent a diagnostic list, but if you do recognize many of the symptoms, or recognize your own winter mood fluctuations, then don't ignore it.

It took me an embarrassingly long time to realize that I had SAD, especially as a neuropsychologist. There is a tendency among healthcare professionals to minimize their own health issues because they are clinically focused on others. I was vaguely aware of my SAD symptoms, but I thought I could push through them by staying busy and distracting myself, so

I didn't stop to properly explore or identify them. I mentioned that SAD is often dismissed, and I believe I too dismissed it as a possibility. It might have something to do with the name. Somehow, acknowledging that you feel 'sad' over winter minimizes its seriousness. As we know, winter can be a challenging time of year anyway, and so we have many reasons to hand to explain away feeling below par. Due to the temporary nature of SAD, by the time I realized something was wrong and made a medical appointment to seek help, I began to feel better and so would cancel it.

I couldn't ignore it for ever, though, and after several years of these feelings recurring, I finally realized that there was an element of my winter mood that I couldn't distract myself out of, or avoid, through sheer will and busyness. I learned to understand SAD and the role it was playing in my futile battle against winter. In fact, SAD *was* my main battle against winter. Once I managed that, the world of winter looked very different.

It is common for human beings, with fluctuating brain chemistry and hormones, to experience episodes of depression and anxiety. These are sometimes called the 'common colds' of the mind, and roughly 1 in 6 will experience symptoms of one or the other or both at any given time.[1] I never attributed my low mood to one particular season. When I was in my mid-twenties, I experienced a few major life events, including a bereavement, which happened across autumn and winter. When the next couple of winters rolled around and I felt rubbish, tearful and depressed, I put it down to memories and associations of grief and sad times. But more winters arrived, and it never improved. In fact, things got distinctly worse.

Far from being sporadic episodes, I was now depressed for four to five months at a time, with very little reprieve, from October onwards. At about the same time, I noticed that I was really responsive to the weather, in a way that I hadn't been when I was younger. When we had a bright sunshine-and-blue-sky kind of day, I felt amazing. I'd be singing in the car and dancing around the kitchen. Then the weather would turn and plummet into dark grey depths, and it would drag my mood down with it.

Put simply, I was happier in the sunshine and sadder in the gloom. I still didn't really think I had SAD because blaming the weather for all-encompassing depression felt far too simple. But I also knew that this wasn't a typical depressive episode. I was frustrated and annoyed that my clinical background and expertise weren't helping me. I think I was also scared to admit that it was something out of my control. I mean, I can't do anything about the weather, so I wanted another explanation. One I could fix. Then, through my work, I was updating a document that required me to research SAD, and I felt as though someone had looked inside my brain. I finally knew what was wrong. Anyone who has sought a diagnosis will know that lightbulb moment. The click. The final piece slotting into place. The relief.

It took me some time to adjust. Was it really something as simple as the weather? Could sunshine really be the answer to something so drastic, so all-encompassing, so debilitating? I needed to find out.

I briefly considered a relocation to somewhere sunny abroad, then remembered I worked in public-sector healthcare, where the salary doesn't really run to exotic relocations, so I did some research and bought myself a sunrise lamp instead. If you haven't seen one, it is a small bedside lamp that utilizes a daylight bulb and slowly imitates a sunrise, getting brighter over a period of half an hour or so. The idea is that you wake up gently and naturally to 'daylight', instead of frantically shutting off the aggressive tones of your alarm clock in the pitch black.

I will never forget that first morning. I woke up smiling, stretching and thinking, 'Gosh, what a beautiful day!' and I felt good. Really good. Of course, I then walked through to my kitchen to discover that it was actually still pitch black outside but, for some reason, that didn't matter. The positive influence had already taken effect, and I felt amazing. I had a bounce in my step for the first time in months and, most importantly, I wasn't crying. It's hard to explain the despair you have to feel to start every morning crying, but those who have any experience with SAD or depression will be familiar with it. To wake up feeling good, happy, dry-eyed and positive about the day ahead was incredible.

My sunrise lamp was also a game changer at bedtime. I set up the sunset function, designed to mimic the naturally fading light of sunset, and clambered into bed with my book. I started reading, then yawning and, many hours later, I woke up to find my book on my face after I had dropped off into the deepest, most restorative sleep I'd had for a long time. Heavenly.

There isn't a good scientific reason why some people get SAD and others don't, which, as a neuropsychologist, I find intensely frustrating. I want an area of the brain to pin the problem on and start fixing. However, what we do know is that SAD is more than your average 'winter blues'. Whilst it is normal for everyone to experience short-term dips in mood, particularly at this time of year, SAD is more pervasive and prolonged. According to the Seasonal Affective Disorder Association (SADA), SAD is a major depressive episode that occurs in relation to specific seasons of the year and can last up to five months. That's nearly half the year spent battling significant depression. It can be daunting to read this information, but I also found it hugely normalizing. As a psychologist who knew all the tips for managing mood, I didn't understand why my strategies for treating depression weren't working for me. To realize that I wasn't using the right strategies and that my low mood was down to real and, comfortingly, treatable SAD gave me hope.

The treatments for SAD are fairly straightforward and non-invasive. Light therapy is the number one recommended solution. In addition to my sunrise/sunset alarm clock, I invested in a SAD lamp, which I sit in front of for at least 60 minutes every morning and sometimes in the afternoon as well. I don't have to sit there doing nothing in that time; my SAD lamp sits on my desk whilst I work, just to the side of my computer screen. The difference it makes is felt immediately. I feel more balanced, stronger, better able to cope, less emotional and overall lighter.

Vitamin D supplementation throughout autumn and winter is also recommended, but lack of vitamin D is not often recognized as an issue. The UK government introduced guidelines from Public Health England in 2016, but a survey by the British Nutrition Foundation revealed that 49% of adults are still unaware of the guidelines.[2] Vitamin deficiency overall is really downplayed in our healthcare system and we need to be more aware of the impacts of low levels of vitamin D on our health. In the UK, 1 in 6 of us has a vitamin D deficiency[3] and as many as 1 in 4 experience this in the US.[4] The symptoms can range from fatigue, insomnia and depression to bone and muscle aches, hair loss and poor immunity. The recommendation is that we supplement from October through to March. We are advised that although a balanced diet can give us most of the nutrients we need, vitamin D is an exception. Our main source is UV exposure from sunlight on skin, and there are relatively few rich dietary sources of vitamin D.[5] This means that in winter, with less sun exposure, it is challenging to top up our vitamin D levels naturally.

A simple blood test can reveal your vitamin D levels and highlight any issues. Your healthcare practitioner can advise you on the levels you need to supplement and what is a safe range for you, so it is always worth consulting them before starting any supplementation. A vitamin D supplement from October to March has become a routine part of my winter regime and has worked wonders for my mood.

Light therapy and vitamin D don't stop me experiencing

the normal ups and downs of mood that come with being human, but I no longer suffer endless months of depression. SAD was a winter companion I did not wish for, nor would I wish it on anyone else. If you are feeling SAD, do not dismiss it. So little is known or shared about SAD and, as previously described, it can be minimized as just 'feeling a bit sad'. Take heart, courage and confidence from knowing that some simple solutions exist to help you feel more *you* over winter. For me, overcoming my SAD was a huge part of my journey towards loving winter again. Once I'd separated out winter from the mood I felt during it, that changed how I felt about the season and how I approached it. I still have to manage my SAD every autumn and winter; it hasn't simply gone away. But the *battle* is over. Winter and I can get along once more. Minimizing my SAD symptoms makes space for other, more positive emotions in winter, which is a wonderful gift.

Normal winter blues and when to seek help

The UK National Health Service (NHS) estimates that 1 in 15, nearly 7% of the population, will experience SAD.[6] The American Psychiatric Association (APA) predicts around 5% of adults in the US experience SAD, typically lasting for 40% of the year.[7] These statistics may seem relatively low to explain the collective slump in mood that is common throughout the darker autumn/winter months. There are other factors at play, from our mindset and thoughts about winter to the way our brains are wired, and these are all important to consider. But we also have 'winter blues'.

Mental health experts at the US National Institutes of Health advise that 'winter blues' is a general term, not a medical diagnosis. Winter blues are common and present as more mild than serious. They should typically resolve in a fairly short amount of time.[8] As mentioned, winter blues are different to full-blown SAD. Health practitioners are in agreement that it is normal to experience a dip in mood that lasts a couple of weeks, often occurring after the festivities of the holiday season have concluded and life returns to normal.

This is the biggest defining factor between winter blues and the more serious SAD. If you feel low for a few weeks over winter but quickly bounce back, it is likely that you are experiencing winter blues. Winter blues may not carry the severity or longevity that SAD does, but they still need to be considered. There is a natural dip in mood in winter and, like all fluctuations, we can lessen the impact by preparing for it.

The light therapy and vitamin D strategies, combined with a focus on good mental health practices, such as sleeping, eating well and exercising, are likely to rapidly improve our mood and dissipate winter blues. It is worth noting at this point that a couple of weeks after the festive holiday season has concluded is also the time when we begin to have more daylight and more exposure to vitamin D. Nature experiences a slight uplift in energy, and so do we. Also, many of us start exercising in January, thanks to some fairly ambitious New Year's resolutions.

We experience an increase in endorphins and oxytocin and all the other mental health benefits that come with being more active. Therefore, the timing of this pick-up in our mood is not wholly surprising when looked at within the wider context.

If you cannot shift your mood or you are feeling low for longer than a few weeks, then it is worth considering whether you are experiencing SAD and seeking the advice of an expert health practitioner. Whether sad or SAD, do not dismiss your winter mood. There is so much that can be done to lift and support it, and winter is the perfect season to provide those solutions.

Chapter 3:
A shift in mindset

Our mindset going into winter influences our wellbeing and overall mood. Here in the UK, we are told that the third Monday in January is the most depressing day of the year, so much so that it has been nicknamed 'Blue Monday'. In both clinical and corporate settings, I have seen individuals express a real dip in mood on Blue Monday. I've seen companies provide extra help and support for the day to boost people's mood and cushion the impact.

If you have ever felt affected by Blue Monday, then I'm not sure how to tell you this . . . it isn't a real thing. It's a myth. The term was first coined in 2005 by psychologist Cliff Arnall as part of a PR stunt by the travel company Sky Travel, designed to sell more holidays. Arnall later admitted that he used pseudo-science and that the date of Blue Monday had no scientific basis. Arnall has since apologized for making January appear far more depressing and joyless than it actually is.[1]

Whilst we can't deny that Blue Monday is a scam, we have

to admit it's a successful one. Backed by our own 'evidence' of gloomy weather, post-Christmas debt and failed New Year's resolutions, we have unwittingly made sense of it and wholly bought into it, coming to believe it is scientifically sound. But it's not. It is, however, a beautiful example of how susceptible we are to being primed to feel a certain way. By believing that Blue Monday is the most depressing day of the year, we are *primed* to feel our most depressed on that day. Would you really look forward to January, or winter as a whole, knowing that the supposedly most depressing date of the entire year resided in it? Probably not.

The importance of mindset cannot be overestimated and this is why we need to start to think differently about winter. If we continue to approach winter telling ourselves that it will be hard, then it will be. It is not the seasons that need to change in order for us to be happier; it's our approach to them. Winter invites us to improve our mood. Winter offers us the encouragement to plan, plot, build and grow our ideas. A space to nourish ourselves and consider what *we* want. It's often the reset we need to put ourselves back into the centre of our own lives. We just need to be open to that invitation.

A reflective winter

The word 'solstice' comes from the Latin words for 'sun' and 'stationary' or 'stopped'. It's also interpreted as the sun standing still. This is because, for the first few days following the winter solstice, the sun will begin its journey north, meaning the days become longer. However, the changes are extremely subtle at first, and so the sun is said to be 'standing still'.

In this sense, the winter solstice is a celestial reminder to stand still. To pause. To reflect. To keep our changes small and subtle. To move forwards, but oh so gently and softly; this isn't the time for dazzling brightness. Yet, what do we do in the days following the solstice? Crash into the festivities of the holiday season, hold big noisy gatherings, eat and drink too much and then put ourselves under huge pressure to start ambitious new plans and goals. Winter offers us an opportunity to sit quietly and reflect, but all too often we resist.

I do understand this resistance. Society tells us that this is a time to be noisy and social. A time for high-energy resolutions and the kickstarting of new routines. But what if it wasn't? What if there was a softness and a gentleness to our winter months? What if we accepted the invitation to slow down?

There is no doubt that I am driven to reflect more during winter. I am more thoughtful, I am slower to make decisions, I am more exacting in my actions and everything is a little more considered. There is a purpose in this slow-down, and how I view it is up to me. I can see it as mindful or I can see it as frustrating. Useful or limiting. My mindset around my behaviour determines how I react to it and the conclusions that I draw from it.

A winter slow-down is designed not to frustrate us, but rather to support us. It is a time to reflect on what has served us really well and what we want to change for the year ahead. It is a time to revisit journeys we have made and wander down their paths, looking around, observing. It is less harsh, less critical, less energized than marching through our to-do lists. That is for more frenetic summer energy. Winter is a time to sit beside our aims, goals, thoughts and ambitions and reflect on where we are, what we need and where we want to go. Winter is the season to open up the map, look at where we want to head and plan our journey. If we accept winter's gentle invitation to pause and reflect, it may be the most productive season of our whole year.

A challenge to our winter mood is that reflection without direction can lead to depression. Our thoughts can turn to self-criticism and negativity. Without guidance, our winter brain can run through imaginary arguments and relive painful memories. Our brain naturally runs through the negatives in order to protect us from harm, so whilst it is well-meaning, it can make quiet reflective time really painful. This is where avoidance kicks in. We sense that our brain is pulling us into this period of deeper, more thoughtful connection with ourselves; we anticipate the pain, and we resist it. We push on through. We stay busy and rush around. We run away from our mind.

The winter blues we experience can happen when, driven indoors by poor weather and cancelled plans, we are forced to confront our own suppressed thoughts, and we don't feel ready to do so. What if we changed that? What if rather than feeling forced into reflection unprepared, we deliberately invited reflection in? Instead of being threatened by our thoughts and emotions, we playfully explored them, much like a child rambling through a forest, stopping to examine a tree root or delighting in an unexpected flower or conker? The forest of our mind can seem intimidating, dark and forbidding, but when we choose to reflect with curiosity and compassion, our thoughts and experiences become a propitious playground.

The aim is not to avoid what might be painful. There will be ups and downs throughout our seasons, and it is important to gently reflect on both. But we want to make sure we aren't viewing everything through a challenging, confronting or critical lens. We need balance in our reflections and we need to manually introduce that balance to counter our brain's natural skew towards the negative. Our brains are natural pessimists, but they are capable of positive thoughts and reflections. We just need to give them a helping hand by deliberately weaving that positivity into our inner narrative.

The key to winter reflection is to avoid harsh judgement; it's not a good time for critique. Rather, this is a time to take stock and observe. Imagine stuffing your feelings into a bag that you carry around everywhere with you. Eventually, that bag is going to get heavy, and you may struggle to find the good in there when it is buried underneath feelings of negativity and doubt. Although we may not want to see these negative emotions, we have to give them the opportunity to leave us, and that means taking them out of the bag. If we never give space to these feelings, we can never let them go. Winter is the perfect opportunity to let the difficult gently fade away. Doing this means we enter the new season with space in our bags, ready to gather all the new experiences and feelings waiting for us. It is a time to unburden in a soft, exploratory way.

It is particularly useful to have questions to guide our reflection. Whenever our brains drift, reflective questions ground us and refocus our thoughts in a more boundaried and balanced way.

How to plan for the more reflective times and days

As with everything in winter, we should reflect with intention. I recommend taking some time to create an easeful space where you can gift yourself some uninterrupted time to think (see Chapter 5, page 54, on creating your own winter retreat). Consider the following questions to guide your winter reflections. It may be that you put a chunk of time aside to answer these questions all in one go. Or perhaps you pick one at random, meditate on that question for a few minutes and then make notes on your thoughts and reflections.

Journalling is a powerful reflective tool, and I am a big believer in getting thoughts out of our heads and onto a page. It is really useful to read our reflections back, perhaps reading them out loud in order to hear our own thoughts. It changes how we interact with them. We can read back our reflections and be surprised and proud at how well we handled a situation that at the time felt messy and out of control, or proud of simply coming through it.

When we reflect on 'the previous year', it can be tempting to think that we must follow the calendar year, and therefore, all this reflection needs to happen around 31 December, ready to start afresh in the new year. However, as we learned in the first chapter, we know that we can rework our year to suit us. We can dip into these reflections throughout the whole season of winter and space them throughout the season, revisiting them whenever feels helpful.

 Activity: Reviewing and renewing reflections

Reviewing: Reflective questions and journal prompts for the past year

1. What word would you use to describe yourself this last year?
2. What are your highlights from the last year?
3. What have you learned over the last year, e.g. a new skill, new information or a realization about yourself or others?
4. How have you nurtured yourself this year?
5. What are you most proud of this year?
6. Who smiled this year because of you?
7. What did you question this year?
8. What of this year (memories, experiences, moments of courage or strength) do you want to package up and carry forward to next year?

9. What can you leave behind in this year?
10. What can you say thank you to this year for?
11. What is the image that best captures/encapsulates this year for you?
12. Who or what did you love this year?
13. What made you laugh out loud this year?
14. What did you lose this year?
15. What did you gain this year?
16. If you were to go back in time, sit down and have a cuppa with the past you of one year ago, what would you want them to know about the year they are about to experience?

Renewing: Reflective questions and journal prompts for the year ahead

1. I am setting my intention for the coming year. This year will be _____
2. How do I want to feel this year?
3. How will I support my health and happiness this year?
4. Who do I want around me this year?
5. What is one project that I would be so excited to complete this year? What is going to be the first step I take towards it?
6. What am I most excited for this year?
7. What is potentially my biggest challenge this coming year? How will I support myself through it?
8. What am I planning for myself this year?

9. What is important to me this year?
10. In what way would I like to grow this year?
11. How do I want to handle challenges this year?
12. What can I stop carrying this year?
13. What would make me happy this year?
14. Who around me shares my vision and ambition for the year ahead?
15. How will I make space for reflection this year?
16. What gift from this season can I carry through the rest of the year?

Deliberately reflecting on our past year and the year ahead of us allows us to channel and process our thoughts without getting stuck in rumination. This makes reflection a nourishing and welcoming safe space. Return to these questions whenever you feel reflective or need grounding in your thoughts.

Wallow like a hippo

Sometimes, no matter the reflections we actively engage in, we can be met with challenges to our mood and our happiness. We will experience ups and downs in all seasons, including winter. Whilst this may not sound like the most evidence-based psychological advice you'll ever hear, I encourage you to be a hippo. Whatever you are dealing with, whether that's being ill and run-down, feeling low in energy or mood, or just feeling a bit off, I urge you to act like a hippo. Let me explain.

Have you ever seen a hippo wallow in mud? They really go for it. There is no skirting around the edge, trying to avoid getting dirty. They wade right into that mud bath, dunk themselves down, getting every single inch of themselves covered in gloriously thick and sticky mud. You can see them revel in it: they roll in it, they play in it, they are absolutely *in* that mud. Then they get out, let the mud dry, shake it off and move on. That's what we need to do with our mood. Rather than desperately trying to avoid the mud bath of our mood, we need to get in and wallow. We need to roll around and embrace that mud. We need to cover ourselves in it. But, much like the hippo, we don't unpack and live there. Instead, we wallow, then we climb out and shake the mud off.

'Wallowing' has a bad reputation. We see it as self-pitying or indulgent, and many of us resist, pushing through tiredness or low mood, endlessly trying to avoid the mud. But here's the thing: we can't. We end up in the mud regardless.

When I was younger, prioritizing career ambition ahead of my health, I used to push through head colds. I remember glibly washing down ibuprofen and paracetamol with whatever caffeine was within reach because I 'didn't have time to be ill'. I honestly felt this was the best way to keep going, but I noticed that my colleagues would get over their colds really quickly whilst mine were still hanging around two weeks later. I was completely lost as to what they were doing that I was not doing, until it dawned on me. They wallowed. If they felt ill, they went to bed. They stopped, they rested, they relaxed. Whilst I pushed through, sticking to my rigid routines, they had a lie-in and gave their bodies the much-needed rest that they were asking for. They wallowed, and as a result, they climbed out of their mud so much quicker than I did.

One Saturday, nearly 10 years ago, I was forced to wallow. I caught a cold at the same time as hurting my ankle, so I had to stay inside and not do much. I gathered all my snacks and blankets and stayed put for the whole day, only getting up for bathroom breaks or to refill my cup of tea. I really resented the 'waste' of my weekend, but I woke up on the Sunday feeling better. My congested sinuses were clearer, my mood was brighter and I had more energy. My 'wasted' Saturday had actually been a much-needed recharge. I had batted away a cold in 48 hours, instead of dragging it out for two weeks. I was converted to wallowing.

If you are reading this and thinking, like I used to, 'I don't have time to be ill,' then believe me when I tell you, if you don't make the time, your body will force you to make the time. Things will pass as quickly as you choose to act, so pay attention to your health and act quickly.

I often fought low mood with the same ferocity as one would a wild tiger. I wrestled with it, attacked it, refused to give in to it, often damaging myself in the process. Until I decided to wallow. The next time I felt low and fed up, I thought to myself, 'OK, I am fed up today,' and didn't try to force myself to feel better or be positive. I just let myself feel fed up, and I noticed that by the early evening I felt better.

Now, I am not saying that wallowing is a magical cure for all ills, but it certainly prevents mental and physical challenges from being unnecessarily dragged out for an extended period of time. We can worry that once we give into a mood, it will overwhelm or define us but, much like the hippo, when we wallow, we don't stay there. We get in and we get out. This approach in winter allows us to follow our energy and really connect to what we need. The slowing down, the invitation to rest, the chance to refocus on ourselves . . . winter offers all of this and provides us with the gift of time to regroup. We don't need to lie around doing nothing; wallowing can be as simple as allowing ourselves to be in an authentic mood state, rather than skirting around the edges. If you're not feeling great, whether physically or mentally, then winter is the perfect time to get in the mud. So, I encourage you to be a hippo: wallow and then climb out and shake that mud off.

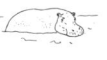 **Activity: How to be a hippo and not get stuck in the mud: a five-step guide**

Step 1: Give in to your wallow completely. Tune in to your mood, accept it and fully embrace being in it.
Step 2: Set a time limit without expectations. Don't pressure yourself with 'I'm giving myself an hour, then

I'm going to snap out of this' but do have a tangible limit to your wallow. If you give yourself two days, spend the first day in the intense wallow and then use the remaining time for the gentle climb out of the mud.

Step 3: Have your ultimate comforts around you. I recommend keeping a wallow box somewhere safe for such occasions. This can hold your favourite chocolate bar, book, notebook, tea/coffee, etc. All the goodies you need without having to think or find the energy to gather them.

Step 4: Plan your escape. Once you have been wallowing for a good few hours, grab a pen and notepad and start planning. Make a list of all the things you want to do once you feel more like yourself. Please note that, importantly, this is *not* a to-do list of all the chores and actions you feel guilty about not doing. If you're going to focus on and get anxious about all the stuff you should be doing, then, in all honesty, just do them because that's not wallowing; that's worrying. Rather, the list you want to write is a list detailing how you will feel and who you want to be once you're out of the mud. This list reminds your brain that this too shall pass and that this is a temporary state; you won't feel like this for ever.

Step 5: Begin your climb out. Choose one achievable item on your list and begin your climb out. Perhaps you'll start with something simple like putting fresh linen on your bed. Before you go to sleep, highlight two more items from your list that you will do tomorrow. When you wake up, ease into your day with your list and know that you have begun your ascent out of the mud. Your energy and attitude are still gentle towards yourself, but you know the mud is drying and you're about to shake it off.

That is how to wallow, and whilst we can wallow in any season, winter, with its invitation to slow down and be gentle with ourselves, is the perfect wallowing season.

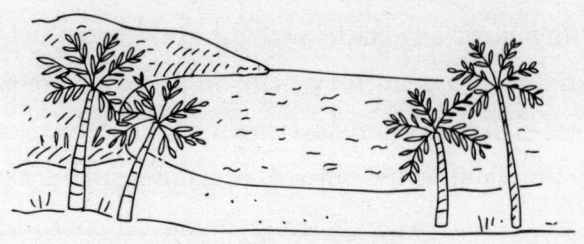

Chapter 4:
Embracing a winter break

As the 1963 Cliff Richard song tells us, 'We're all going on a summer holiday.'¹ I must admit, I have never quite understood why it is that when the weather is most likely to be warm, sunny and inviting, we choose to leave it and go somewhere else.

We grit our teeth through winter weather and wait until the summer months only to then go and bake in hotter climes, all whilst the sun shines at home. The disappointment of going abroad only to receive WhatsApp photos of sunny back gardens and barbecues from home is real. Despite this, the Tripadvisor Summer Travel Index (2023) found that, of the 81% of Brits planning holidays between the months of June and August, more than two-thirds will go abroad. Meanwhile, I am definitely one of the 31% who plan to enjoy warmer weather at home over the summer months.² For many years now I have chosen to take my main holiday in the winter months. Whether I choose to chase the sunshine and experience different winters across the world or embrace a retreat at home, a winter break is a game changer.

I know what you may be thinking here. 'Hang on a minute. This is a book about the gifts of winter, and you are telling me to run away and escape them?!' Actually, I'm not. I encourage you to take a break to be *in* winter, no matter whether that's at home (see Chapter 5, page 54, on creating your winter retreat) or further afield. Far from encouraging you to escape winter, I am encouraging you to take a break and truly experience winter.

My own winter breaks vary. Sustainability and climate considerations, alongside financial ones, influence my holiday decisions. But I do always take a winter break, whether at home or away. My first proper holiday in winter – rather than just the 'my office is closed between Christmas and New Year' enforced time off – changed my entire year in the most positive and wonderful way, and I've never looked back. The first time I had a sunny winter break, I went East and travelled to Thailand. I'd never been, I had no idea what to expect, and it felt truly bizarre to be packing a swimsuit and flip-flops whilst wearing a Fair Isle jumper and polishing off the remains of the Christmas cake. When I arrived, I messaged my mum to let her know that I was there safely and she replied, 'It is 2 degrees here – enjoy every second!' I knew then that this was the time of year when I wanted to travel. I was never again going to seek adventures abroad in the summer months.

Initially, I misunderstood the benefit of my winter break. I thought, 'Aha! I've cracked it! I just need to go away every winter!' I was so convinced that this was the answer to my

SAD that I became quite fearful of coming home, fearful that a rushing recurrence of SAD symptoms would prove too much for me. But it didn't happen. It wasn't about the sunshine; it was the total alignment of that break with my energy levels. Stopping at a time when I needed to stop. Refuelling at a time when all my resources were low. Winter that year invited me to pause, and for the first time, I did. Now, you could be forgiven for thinking that this was the effect of warmth and sunshine, and there is no denying the perk of extra vitamin D during the winter months. However, during the second Covid lockdown, I continued my tradition of taking a week or two off at the beginning of the year, even though there was nowhere to go. I walked. I sang. I cooked. I danced. I read. I also ventured out and spent time *in* winter. I made a point of getting outside, no matter the temperature, and something magical happened. I felt good. Really good.

How would you feel if you started winter with a break? When you review your year, is now the perfect time for some rest and relaxation? Would your year look different if you started it with a pause? I was very aware that my winter break would be my big holiday of the year and wondered if I would regret using up my annual leave in January. I am a planner by nature, and part of my joy in a holiday is having it to look forward to. I worried that once my January holiday had passed, the rest of the year would feel interminable in length. However, quite the opposite happened. I felt invigorated and reflective. I wrote page after page in my journal.

I had space for creativity and became excited as my plans and ambitions for the year ahead crystallized. I also realized the impact of physically moving more. I trekked and explored and wandered during a time that typically can feel stagnant and bloated following the festivities. I planned and organized. I wrote and listed. I paused. I breathed. I took a break. That's when I realized: this isn't about the sunshine or an exotic destination. It's about matching winter energy to get exactly what you need.

I really encourage you to rethink your holiday planning and consider a winter break. If you are constrained by the school holidays, research shows that it's cheaper to travel in winter than in summer, with an average saving of nearly £300 per person.[3] This can help combat the shamefully blatant parent tax that holiday companies force on families. With summer prices excluding so many from the possibility of a break, taking your main holiday in winter can be the solution.

Summer is our high-energy season, and it doesn't require us to take a break. We have nature, daylight and summer foods that help us to be more active, more focused and more driven. The idea of trying to take a break when you have all the energy and oomph of the year piled high in your favour feels counterintuitive, like having a double espresso before bed or putting a full tank of petrol in your car and then not driving anywhere for a few weeks. Winter, by contrast, offers us an invitation to do things differently.

The myth of the trough

I have worked for and with corporations of all sizes and, despite the very varied nature of their core business, they all have one thing in common: the myth of the trough.

Usually, ahead of winter, employees will start talking about the wind-down in the run-up to the festivities. There will be generic conversations in the office or on the shop floor about the upcoming holiday season and the wrapping up and shutting down that will happen before 'everyone goes off on holiday'. However, whilst I have witnessed the peaks countless times, I have yet to experience a trough, especially not in winter.

The push towards achieving more seems endless. The rallying cries to ramp up production, to restructure and reorganize, to 'build back better'. Companies put their employees on a treadmill and continuously press the speed-increase button. Employees are continuously being asked to boost energy, motivation, production and output. Then, just as they find their stride, the pace increases again. And again. And again. Although this clearly isn't sustainable, I have never once witnessed a slowing down. A reduction in tempo. A trough.

Sometimes, long-serving employees will look at each other and say, 'Do you remember when there was a quiet time to balance out these peaks?' On further investigation, it transpires that they are referring to a time many years, sometimes decades ago. We need to be mindful that, far from being a wind-down period at work, winter can be one of the busiest times of the year, and the way organizations work can add to the pressure.

At the exact same time that we are meant to be winding down, we are often also taking part in end-of-year reviews and personal evaluations. We can be under huge pressure to get purchase orders from suppliers and quickly push things over the line, ahead of the start of the new year. Winter remains so busy at work partly due to 'winding down for the holidays', even if this is only a perceived wind-down. We feel an urgency to get everything done, and there can be a horribly dissatisfying and unfinished feel to the year if projects carry over to January. We can also experience an increase in demand but a decrease in support. We've probably all had the experience of relying on others to get a project over the line, only to receive their out-of-office auto-reply in mid-December.

Not only that but in line with your end-of-year review, you may be asked to think about your professional objectives for the year ahead. Where are we supposed to find the headspace for reflection, planning and ambition during this increasingly pressurized and stressful period? All in all, you are being asked to finalize, wrap up, evaluate and sign off on work at a point in the year when your workload doesn't seem to lessen (has no one told it about the mythical trough?). Not forgetting that personal pressure is often also at an all-time high. With the festivities around the corner and all the chaos of planning, ordering and scheduling that comes with them, we are often at peak stress. All of this clashes against a season that is asking for something very different. It's asking for a break. Not just from your work but, as rude as this sounds, also from your colleagues.

Clashing with colleagues

As we enter winter, our bodies respond to the changing environment around us and our brains seek a change. Having done all the hard work and thinking during the higher-energy months, our brains are ready to settle into the restorative, contemplative nature of winter. This is a direct contrast to the push push push attitude of those around us. Coupled with additional social pressures, such as the office get-together and the pre-holiday catch-ups with colleagues who suddenly want your time, energy and attention, it can feel too much. These meet-ups take on an inexplicable urgency ahead of the holidays ('but we *must* meet up before Christmas'), and this can make for a very hectic time of year. We carry a heavier cognitive load, trying to balance demands from all sides, and our stress response becomes heightened. We can feel moodier, snappier and more emotional, and this means that the colleague demanding that report, or the manager who wants you to boost production, is not just annoying, but actively going against the way that your brain wants to work. Additional noise, pressure and stress can make us feel crowded and overwhelmed, but it is not that we are not coping well; it is that we *have* coped well. Now nature is advising us to be gentle and restorative, which might not align with Clive from accounts wanting that report *now*.

Winter workloads

Whilst winter workloads can feel very overwhelming and pressured, we actually do a lot better than we think. It is probably no surprise that we are less productive in winter. However, we are only *slightly* less productive, with research showing we complete 7.2% of our yearly tasks in January, 7.6% in February and 8.3% in March.[4] An equal divide across 12 months would mean 8.33% of tasks achieved each month, so winter does not see a dramatic decrease. However, the *feel* of this achievement and productivity is what differentiates winter from other seasons. Winter is such a re-energizing time, as long as we make some minor helpful tweaks and pay attention to clashes. If we do, then winter will be infinitely easier. We can accommodate the slight drop in productivity by adjusting our planning, in and out of work, to accommodate it. We can also adjust our work and social diaries, our beliefs about when we must holiday and manage our own expectations. These small mindset and practical shifts release the pressure and the battles we face when working in winter.

One of the mindset shifts we can make around winter breaks is the expectation around a winter break itself. People sometimes say to me, 'There's no point taking a break in winter because it's not nice outside.' I would argue that this is exactly why it is the *perfect* time for a break. There is definitely a mindset blocker that suggests we can't go anywhere or do anything in winter, and it prevents us from taking a break.

And yet, why commute in the dark and try to continue daily life when it is clearly the perfect time *not* to do those things? Even a short break, a reprieve, a time to do nothing can support you through winter. Just as during the pandemic, when more than 57 million days of annual leave went unclaimed, with 48% of Britons surveyed considering it 'pointless' to take a break as they couldn't go abroad,[5] we rarely take a break in winter. We need to change our mindset about that.

Contrary to the popular opinion that people have simply run out of paid time off by the time winter rolls around, a 2023 YouGov survey found that 50% of working adults in the UK do not take their full annual leave allocation.[6] This is in spite of nearly 79% of those same adults surveyed reporting that taking a break is good for their mental health. This means that there is plenty of annual leave to be taken at the beginning of the year. In my experience, there is less competition and therefore more chance of it being agreed with work as well. It is a very different experience to come back to work knowing that you have a January/February break scheduled and that you are creating your own trough, your own pressure-release valve in your working year. Our bodies are telling us that we need to adjust our sleep and working patterns, yet work persists in telling us we need to get up at the same time and get moving. It's hard to get out of bed in the winter months for a reason: we're supposed to be staying put! Taking a break during winter months, even a short one, allows you to reset and reconnect with the natural rhythms around you. It is an opportunity to take a break from the battle. To let go of expectations that literally clash with the fibres of your being.

Granted, not everyone has the privilege of paid time off, and those that do may be anchored to specific times of the year due to school holidays and childcare arrangements, etc. However, those who can take the time off should consider it. Our traditional pattern of working all year, having a break in summer and asking our brains to push through seasonal changes is failing us. We are simply not designed to push when the world around us is demanding a hush, and so we have to balance our work needs accordingly. There is no trough any more. There is no dip. There is no quiet. It is a myth. If we want to experience a slow-down, a pause, a trough, then we need to be the ones to create it.

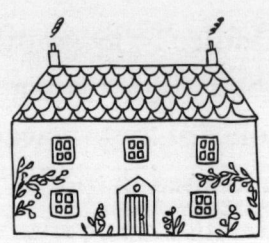

Chapter 5:
A winter retreat at home

Cosmognosis is the instinctive force that tells an animal when and where to migrate, directing them to follow the path that will serve them best over winter. In the lead-up to winter, I feel my own metaphorical cosmognosis kick in, guiding me to my very own hibernaculum, my winter refuge, somewhere to retreat to during the winter months. I don't have far to travel because I create my winter retreat at home. I make small, energetic shifts in my surroundings, which allow my home to become a place with no pressure, expectation or obligation for the entire season. My winter retreat is a place to simply *be* with winter.

Creating a winter retreat

I started creating my winter retreats after stumbling across an article about creating a yoga retreat at home. I hadn't had a holiday for about five years at this point and was dreaming of a break that I couldn't afford. The article proposed a seven-day retreat and offered different ways to start each day. It listed daily rituals to take part in, varied yoga practices to try and new recipes for food and drinks that could be enjoyed each day. Beyond the basics, it also described different ways of being. Different intentions. Different aims for each day.

It struck me that making some relatively small changes could induce that holiday feeling that I was craving, even though I wouldn't be leaving my own home. It wasn't about travelling thousands of miles, but rather about deciding to act differently and not compromise. The proposed retreat was not a combination of home life and retreat life. There was no suggestion of practising sun salutations whilst the washing machine completed its spin cycle. It was a very deliberate full-week planned retreat, and it included lots of downtime, lots of free time and lots of encouragement to take a break. I decided to follow this approach, but instead of a yoga retreat, I wanted to create a winter retreat.

Breaks where we achieve very little can be challenging in a society that tells us we must hustle or that hobbies are only worthwhile when resulting in Instagram-worthy outputs. However, we are not performing in life, we are living it. There is no standing ovation at the end and we need to release the pressure to have everything approved by other people. We don't need to showcase how and what we are achieving. We don't need to be achieving at all.

A soul-nourishing break could, ironically, be our most productive time of the year because that's when we support our body and brain and connect with what we need the most. It may be that a winter retreat where we do nothing but read, relax, meditate, reflect and breathe is exactly what our body is asking for. Imagine the satisfaction of having such a retreat without needing to leave the house. We have lost the art of relaxation. In a world that is so connected and busy and chaotic, we have forgotten the power in a pause, and far from being relaxing, an absence of 'doing' can feel disconcerting. In order to embrace a winter retreat, we need to escape the binds and expectations of productivity. This is not time off to *do* anything. It's time off. Time off responsibility. Time off domesticity. Time off. Treat it like a holiday. You *are* on holiday. A week would be ideal, but if that really is too much to manage, or you have dependents and/or responsibilities that can't be paused, then start with morning retreats. Take yourself for a long walk, watch a movie, read a chapter with a cuppa, dance to your favourite playlist. The point is deliberate time off your normal routine and, as my dad always says, a change is as good as a rest. Also bear in mind that one week is less than 2% of your year. If you are getting no other downtime or break in your year, then at-home retreats can be rebalancing, re-energizing and reinvigorating.

Breaks at home do need some management. It is hard to switch out of 'busy' mode, and some uninterrupted time at home can present a to-do list that you have been meaning to get to for months. Now is not the time to sort cupboards or get a jump on spring cleaning. We have to protect our retreat time with boundaries. We can always use a physical cue; it's good for our brains to get into retreat mode by physically doing something different.

We can plan our retreats at home as we would a holiday. We can stock up on all our favourite foods, wear only super-comfy clothes and disengage from our day-to-day routines. Our mindset needs to be 'I'm on holiday', and so whenever we have the idea of 'I could put some washing on' or 'I should look at that bill that just came through the post', we can tell ourselves that we will, but not until after our holiday.

My first at-home winter break was a wonderful week, and the following year a friend of mine did it too, along with her two children, and we wrote each other postcards from our retreat destinations, aka our own homes. I now look forward to my winter retreats with the same anticipation and excitement as I do any other holiday. It is a chance to stop. To break out of mundanity and to reconnect with my home again. This retreat practice means my home stops being simply a roof over my head, a space that I take for granted, and instead becomes a sanctuary. For a whole week, the only purpose of my home is to be a space where I can be safe and happy and relaxed, and I love it for that.

Retreating with others

We all have different requirements for a holiday. Some of us want beaches and bikinis, others want slopes and après ski and others want adventures. Ultimately, what we all want is a break, and a winter retreat at home can be a game changer. A time when we can recharge our batteries and connect with winter's gentle and restorative energy. With a bit of creativity, a winter retreat can be a near-free holiday for all the family from the comfort of your own home. It is a time to be mindfully present in every element of your day. It is the antidote to the busyness, the chaos, the pressure. It is also the perfect solution for a much-needed break from work.

The word 'retreat' often conjures up associations of withdrawing or removing ourselves from others, but this needn't be the case. Creating a winter retreat within your own home provides a space that your entire household can benefit from. Of course, it's fantastic if any other heartbeats in your house want to join you for a retreat day or two, but the likelihood of you all wanting to relax and restore in the same way, at the same time, is remote. By creating a winter retreat, you are creating spaces for your household to retreat *to*, where you can be together and engage in cosy activities or where you can experience the companionship of winter as you sit quietly together.

A seasonal space

The changes you make to your home for a winter retreat will benefit you through the entire season. You can create somewhere to relax and rest, a cosy nook, a place to think. A space to sit quietly or laugh deeply. Creating this type of winter retreat is a way of escaping not winter but the day-to-day burdens of life that can seem heavier when wrapped in a cloak of darkness.

Remember when you were a child and you built a fort? Somewhere exclusively for you and the precious few that you allowed entry to (usually on the production of the correct password or snacks)? Making your home a winter retreat is the adult version of those pillow walls and bedsheet ceilings. The snacks rule still holds true for me too.

My retreat is not somewhere I escape to for just a couple of hours; it runs deeper than that. It is a mindset. It is a totally different vibe. I create a physically different space for winter, with pillows, blankets, thick, soft, fluffy socks, hot tea and biscuits. I light candles and have relaxing music on softly in the background. It is a space where I exhale and sink a little deeper into the softness of the season.

Changing the energy of our homes to support seasonal winter shifts encourages powerful mindset shifts. It is a useful cue for our brains to slow down, reflect, reconsider and adjust to the season. It's good to reflect on our homes in each season, both on what we need and what our homes need. It is a fantastic way to stay aware of and in tune with the shifting patterns of nature.

Simple changes make a big difference. Wellies by the door. Thicker coats, hats, scarves and gloves on the coat hooks, replacing lightweight summer jackets. Changing your home for the season may sound onerous but, in reality, these are five-minute changes that set you up for the whole season, most of which you're likely to complete in autumn. The very small amount of energy you expend to get ready for winter will be recharged by the energy you get back from making the season so much easier for you and your home.

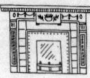 Activity: A home energy audit

What does your home need? Is your home ready for winter?

Take some time to consider your home and what it needs this winter. If you are reading this book in the middle of winter, then consider what may be missing. I encourage you to walk from room to room and think about how you are spending your winter days and if there is anything your home needs in order to support you to 'do' winter better.

Consider the energy of your home as you walk through it. How do you feel in each room? How would you like to feel this winter? What are you facing this winter, and how could your home sustain you through it? What daily gift can your home give you? For example, if you want a warm welcome when you come home, could you keep a basket by the door with a snuggly cardigan and your softest socks? If you want to explore some of the truly beautiful weather and breathe lungfuls of crisp air, could you keep walking boots and cosy gloves to hand?

Some of the changes may be practical. I have two dogs and a cream linen sofa (no, I don't know what I was thinking either), and so thick, washable throws become a feature of our living room during the wetter, muddier seasons. Some of the changes may be pure indulgence.

> Gorgeous scented candles in uplifting fragrances can change the whole mood and energy of a room. Changes don't require expensive shopping trips; they only require thought. You are likely to have everything you need already, you just need to locate and have to hand whatever you need to create your own seasonal retreat space. If you have a little budget to put aside for your retreats, then it's a great opportunity to spoil yourself, even if that's just buying the posh biscuits to dunk in your tea.

Accidental hygge

There are some staples for my winter retreats. Blankets on the sofa to snuggle under. A side table with a coaster for my mug of tea and a notebook and pen for when I feel more reflective and want to capture my thoughts as I let my mind wander unrestrained. TV remote controls are tidied away to put a little bit of friction between me and yet another screen for the day. A perfect winter evening for me is a book, a candle, a cuppa, a snack, a blanket, a snoozing dog or two and some gentle background music.

Although I didn't hear the term until many years after I embraced the concept, the way I set up my home follows the principles and ideas of hygge (pronounced HYOO-guh[1]). Hygge, regarded as a core characteristic of Danish culture, is defined by the Oxford dictionary as 'a quality of cosiness and comfortable conviviality that engenders a feeling of contentment or wellbeing'.[2] That sounds about perfect for a winter retreat to me.

Hygge has become synonymous with 'cosy' and is often linked with an aesthetic, but the feel of hygge runs much deeper. For me, hygge is a mindset, an attitude, an approach. A want and need for life to be softer, gentler, warmer, kinder. It is a break without stopping. Hygge is a way to be, think, feel and immerse yourself. You can sink into hygge as you sink into winter. But hygge is not hibernation. It is not about retreating *away* from the world but rather embracing your world with a new mindset. Hygge is kindness, wrapped in warmth and served in softness.

The defined sense of conviviality is key. Hygge brings a different energy to our socializing and is there to be shared, when we want to. It is easier, less stressful and more friendly, not just to your guests, but to you as the host. Hygge means creating a warm atmosphere and enjoying good times with good people.[3] I created 'hygge days' for my winter calendar to encapsulate the conviviality of hygge, and I highly recommend creating your own hygge days to share with those you love.

A hygge day

The idea of a hygge day started brewing in my mind in my early twenties. As I grew older, I saw how many of my now-adult friends struggled during the festive season. How they were squeezed between everyone else's demands and needs, stressful family dynamics, unreasonable work pressures, etc. I found this acutely sad, especially during a season which pressures us to be happy. I wanted a different approach, and I felt everyone, myself included, deserved some calm in the storm. I wanted to create a day for all those I loved who were feeling overwhelmed by festivities, family events, or just the throes of a new season that they were unprepared for and thus knocked over by. I wanted a space where everyone could just be, with no pressure or obligation. A space to breathe easily. Hence, my hygge days were born.

Put simply, on hygge days, my home becomes a space where people do whatever they want to do. They can arrive when they want, they can stay overnight if they want. They can wear their scruffiest or comfiest clothes or even arrive in their pyjamas; there are no expectations of them. Once here they can read, drink tea, eat, relax, be quiet, have chats and cosy cuppas or sit in silence. One friend arrived on hygge day with her new baby because she needed some adult company whilst breastfeeding. Another arrived with presents that needed sorting and wrapping away from the children. Some of my friends want to turn up and cook, bake, create. Others want to turn up and be fed. There are no real rules to hygge day but although I host, I don't wait on people. The idea isn't that they come and I run around looking after them. The idea is that they have a space to have a winter retreat, a hygge day. They replenish their souls here. I have had four different groups of friends arrive at once and squeeze in together, all doing their own thing, drifting in and out of the kitchen when hungry or thirsty but all revelling in not having to be or do anything that day. I have friends who tell me hygge day is the only day they don't have to be responsible. One friend arrived on hygge day following a tough year, and she slept for hours for the first time in months. Whatever they need, it exists, and the gentle socializing, the togetherness without any pressure, is its own form of winter retreat.

Hygge day provides exactly what you need, whatever that is, whenever you need it. I highly recommend bringing hygge days into your winter and planning your own days of companionship, conviviality and cosiness to boost your sense of winter wellbeing.

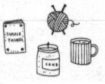

Activity: How to create a hygge day of your own

- **Set your intention.** What do you want to get out of your hygge day? Understanding and setting your intention will help you to establish when and where to create your day.
- **Pick out a time and protect it.** Block out a whole day in your calendar and protect that time as you would a hospital appointment. I'm a big fan of booking off a working day if possible. Weekends can get swallowed up in activities, life admin, children's social commitments, etc., whereas deliberately booking a day off feels like

the ultimate gift to ourselves. It adds a certain air of decadence to the day.

- **Pick a venue.** Choose your location carefully. A hygge day at home means that you have control over your environment, but home isn't relaxing for everyone, especially if we live with other people. If you think you're going to get pulled into life admin, having to find your child's lost PE kit or having to keep explaining yourself in a way that is going to spoil your hygge day, then plan your venue(s) carefully. Case in point, my lovely friend Veronica had explained all about her hygge day to her husband and was most upset when he booked in his car service and assumed she'd deal with it 'because you are off anyway'. Her beautiful and carefully planned day was spent in a draughty garage surrounded by noise and dirt, which was the total opposite of what she had planned. Your hygge day is just for you, to support you in doing exactly what you want to do to nourish your soul, so pick a venue that does exactly that.
- **Pick your company (if any).** If you get very little free time to yourself then it may be that your ultimate hygge day is spent alone. But hygge days can be a gorgeous experience to share with others, you just need to be careful who you choose. You need to be aligned in your intentions for the day. If you turn up wanting a quiet, relaxing and chilled-out day, and they want to rush through January sales, then you'll be left frazzled.

If you do want company, I recommend setting your intention, plan and venue first, then sharing with others and seeing who aligns. Rather than 'Does anyone want to meet up?' send a message saying, 'I am going to X to do Y because I want to feel Z – would anyone like to join me?' This way, you are going to be aligned with, not resenting whoever you share the gift of your hygge day with.

- **Divide the tasks and prepare.** Whether you are spending your hygge day alone or with others, do all the necessary preparation beforehand. If you want to eat your favourite foods, watch your favourite films and light candles, then make sure you do the food shopping, download the films and have the candles ready to light. You don't want your hygge day derailed in the first hour because you cannot remember your Netflix password.

Hygge beyond the day

Hygge is more than just a day; it is a vibe for the whole season. It influences how we set up our home and the mindset with which we approach winter. Even the preparations for hygge are gentle and non-abrasive. There is no scurryfunging (that last-minute frantic tidying we all do before guests arrive). There is no rushing or sudden anything. It is a meander around our homes. Listening and connecting with the space and asking,

'What does my home need from me, and what do I need from my home?'

What I love about hygge is that it stops winter feeling stagnant. There is deliberate comfort, pause and rest in every element, as well as chatter and connection and joy. It isn't a retreat from the world, but rather a retreat *for* the world. Hygge provides a way of creating and embracing the different energies that arise in winter.

Mindfully aligning your company with your intentions and expressing your needs to ensure those around you can support your goals are fantastic strategies to adopt at any time of year, but especially in winter. There is an invitation in hygge. It is the deeper squeeze of winter's hug, and we can comfortably and softly embrace it.

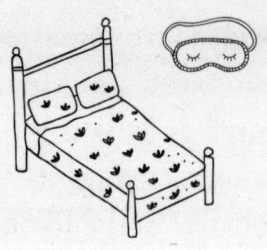

Chapter 6:
A winter bedtime

I love getting into bed. I love the accompanying feelings of safety and security. Getting into bed is a physical out-of-office message we send to the world as we close our eyes on the day. If there is one time of year when bedtime really comes into its own, it's winter. Never is the urge to hurkle-durkle (a gorgeous 19th-century Scottish phrase meaning to lounge in bed long after it is time to get up) as strong as it is in winter. As winter creates a hush, turns down the lights and cools the temperature, there couldn't be a clearer invitation to get into bed, get cosy and get some sleep.

The instinctive need for winter sleep

When I ask people how they feel in December, the most common response is 'tired'. The aptly named 'fall fatigue' describes how our energy levels are depleted in the run-up to winter as our physical, mental and hormonal states change.

These changes are largely associated with reduced sunlight and the resultant impact on serotonin and melatonin production. Although we largely attribute these changes to winter, the reality is that the impacts being felt in our bodies arrive in autumn. The darker mornings start to be really noticeable from October onwards here in the UK, and the subsequent changes in daily and sleep routines challenge our energy levels. Findings from the Sleep Foundation show that those with SAD will sleep an average of 52.9 minutes less per night in October than they did in September.[1] In the run-up to the coolest season, we experience reduced-quality sleep and will be feeling the consequent impacts. Although autumn may not prove a soporific season, winter delivers, with the majority of adults sleeping more in winter.[2] How we leave autumn will have a significant impact on our energy for the season ahead, and fall fatigue explains why we can feel so tired by the end of the year and why we have an instinctive pull towards more sleep in winter.

As humans, we can look to the rest of the animal kingdom and envy those creatures that hibernate. At the end of a busy year, the thought of eating a big meal and sleeping for months on end is extremely appealing. Although we aren't built for hibernating, the instinctual sense we have that we need more sleep in winter is supported by science. A recent study into the seasonality of human sleep showed significant differences in both sleep type and quality across the seasons.[3] In winter, our sleep latency (the time it takes for us to fall asleep once in bed) is shorter, our total sleep time is greater and we experience both more rapid eye movement (REM) sleep and more slow wave sleep (SWS), also known as deep sleep. Both REM and SWS are essential parts of our sleep repertoire. They support various brain functions, including memory and learning, concentration, maintenance of good mental health and mood regulation, and they strengthen our immune system.

Our sleep patterns change to match what we need throughout the year, and our brain recognizes what we need to feel good through winter. These seasonal variations apply in multiple different environments, including urban areas with high levels of noise and light pollution. In other words, our instinctive need for more sleep goes beyond the environment we live in. There is a deeper part of us, rooted in nature, that craves more sleep in winter. Achieving it, however, can be challenging.

A change in routine

My partner and I rarely argue, but one real point of contention is his alarm clock. He would happily keep the same alarm all throughout the year, which drives me to distraction (and exhaustion!).

Every year, I plead the case that we cannot maintain summer sleeping patterns in winter, nor should we try. It is a repetitive annual argument that I do eventually win. Sadly, not through my immense powers of persuasion (he's a stubborn one), but because biologically it makes sense. My partner benefits from the additional sleep, and household harmony is restored.

It is worth saying we are not talking about a dramatic change in routine, but rather a one-hour temporary seasonal shift, which is very achievable, especially if we stop hitting snooze. Snoozing our alarms is not good for us, as a plethora of research repeatedly supports, but snoozing in winter is particularly jarring to the system. If you currently snooze your alarm multiple times, then, instead, set your alarm for the latest time you can and benefit from the extra much-needed seasonal sleep. This will prevent you from experiencing multiple cortisol 'shots' and aggravating your nervous system at the start of your day. If you're worried that you won't get up, then move your alarm out of snooze reach so you have no choice but to get up. If you know you have multiple alarms, you are likely to ignore the first few. Try having one alarm set at the latest time you want to get up and feel the difference in your energy and mood from the get-go.

A small change in sleep habits could form part of your winter adjustment, allowing you to fully embrace a restful and restorative winter. We can go back to earlier alarms and snoozing (if we must) in higher-energy seasons, but in winter, let's adjust our routine and recharge our batteries, recoup our energy and enjoy more extra-cosy-snuggled-in minutes.

Along the same lines, it's also worth considering if this is really the season for jarring life alterations. Friends and clients tell me that they are going to start a 5am routine or begin pre-work gym sessions, which is amazing if that's what they want to do, but maybe not in winter. The invitation is for *more* rest and if we are making changes to our sleep, then we want to align with the season, not clash against it. We get to make the rules of our year, and New Year's resolutions can begin whenever we want them to. The calendar does not have to dictate our habits.

It can feel challenging to make changes to sleep routines when we start work at the same time every day or have to complete the school run. As stated in Chapter 1, there are huge benefits in flexing and adapting our living patterns and rewriting our year to align with the seasons. I strongly believe this is something that our schools and workplaces should pay attention to. However, in the absence of a radical societal overhaul, we will struggle to make changes to our morning routines when external schedule pressures remain static. So, if we can't lie in, we must look to the other end of the day. Instead of focusing on the end of sleep, i.e. getting up, we need to focus on the start of sleep and flex our winter bedtime. Winter invites us to go to bed earlier, so what stops us accepting that invitation and eagerly clambering in?

You may have heard of revenge bedtime procrastination (RBP), where adults fight to stay awake because they feel it's 'too early' to go to sleep yet, even when they are exhausted. The Sleep Foundation defines RBP as 'the decision to sacrifice sleep for leisure time that is driven by a daily schedule lacking in free time'.[4] We take 'revenge' on our busy daily schedules, which offer us no leisure or relaxation time. It is as though by staying up later, we are saying 'screw you!' to our crowded diaries and cramming in 'me time', to the detriment of our sleep.

No doubt we have all sacrificed sleep for the sake of a good night out. As an occasional practice, this causes very little harm and any 'damage' can easily be undone by an early bedtime the following night. However, RBP is different. RBP is the continual and prolonged practice of either delaying going to bed by choosing activities that feel more fun or immediately rewarding, such as watching TV, or delaying going to sleep once in bed, an issue exacerbated by the increased use of electronic devices in bed. Neither is good news.

There are three defining factors to RBP:

1. A delay in going to sleep that reduces one's total sleep time.
2. The absence of a valid reason for staying up later than intended, e.g. an external event or illness.
3. An awareness that delaying one's bedtime could lead to negative consequences.[5]

RBP is the ultimate rejection of winter. We are being invited to rest, recover and recharge. Revenge should not feature in our bedtime routine, and ultimately, we only hurt ourselves. If you have noticed a pattern of RBP, then winter is the perfect time to break that habit. William H. McRaven's popular self-help book tells us that the secret to success is to 'Make Your Bed'.[6] When it comes to winter, the secret to success is to Go to Bed!

A winter recharge

In winter, we draw breath and slowly exhale before the awakening rush of spring begins. It makes sense that more sleep is needed during the gentler phase of the year, when the air around us is less electrified with frenetic energy, and we are encouraged to embrace restorative rest.

The importance of sleep is too often defined by the consequences we experience when we aren't getting enough of it. Let's focus instead on what sleep does *for* us, not what a lack of sleep does *to* us. Sleep is so personal, and all of our bodies are different. We are often fed generic data and targets for our sleep that don't represent what we individually may need in order to support our health and happiness. It's important we don't put pressure on ourselves to meet sweeping aims and goals. It's OK if our sleep pattern does not match someone else's, as long as we get the sleep that *we* need. Sleep is the human equivalent of plugging in a charger. We run down our cell batteries during the day and we recharge them whilst we sleep. Sleep replenishes us; ideally, we awake feeling energized and refreshed.

Whilst our sleeping bodies are still, our brains light up with activity. This is largely when all the upkeep, filing, sorting and admin of the brain is done. Imagine an office manager going through files, making sure that they are stored in the right places and labelled correctly. As our winter brains are in a more reflective state, there is more processing to be done, and getting more sleep is useful to complete this. When we sleep more and process more, we awake with a clearer mind and are better able to focus. It's also a good reason not to swipe and scroll before bed. Our brains process every single piece of information that they receive. There is no way to say to your brain, 'Oh, that's just a nonsense reel, don't worry about that one.' Every image and every video we see on social media or the news is processed. If we feel overwhelmed and exhausted, it is likely due to us asking our brains to process input at a rate that it was never designed to. Our brains are working overtime to absorb the lives of thousands of people we will never meet. If you are feeling tired or as though your head is spinning, put down your phone and let your brain catch up for a bit.

Sleep is important for our immune system and healing. Essentially, our bodies use the time when we are asleep to take us into the repair shop and fix us up. Injuries, muscle tears and strains are better able to heal when we are at rest. Sleep is the ideal counterpart to active rest and recovery. Sleep actively boosts our immune system. It helps balance out and prevent the negative impacts of inflammation in the body[7] whilst fortifying and strengthening innate and adaptive immunity. At a time of year when cold and flu season is rife, winter's offer of more sleep is an opportunity to heal and support our health. It's an invitation to take care of ourselves.

A winter sleep challenge

Whilst we can recognize the power and importance of sleep in winter, it doesn't always follow that we will fall asleep easily. A third of adults worldwide struggle with symptoms of insomnia,[8] and it takes its toll. Knowing the importance of sleep, we need to know how to combat these issues so that we can fall into the sleepy embrace of winter.

A well-documented challenge to winter sleep is the skewed production of melatonin, but maybe not in the way that you think. General media has been advising us for years to 'get outside in the morning to aid your melatonin production', but that's misrepresenting how this amazing process occurs. Melatonin is a natural hormone produced by the pineal gland in the brain and released into the bloodstream. When darkness falls, the pineal gland is prompted to start producing melatonin, which makes us feel sleepy and encourages us to fall asleep. Whilst darkness acts as a prompt for melatonin production, daylight acts as a blocker, keeping us feeling awake and alert during the day.

As our daylight hours reduce in autumn and winter and many of us start and end our day in the dark, we lose that prompt for our brains that it is night-time now and so it's time to produce melatonin. This can completely throw our circadian rhythms off and means that we may feel tired and sleepy all day but yet cannot drop off to sleep at night, as we are missing that definitive hit of melatonin. It is for this reason that so much advice in winter is about getting out in the daylight when you can in order to allow your brain to recognize the difference between daytime and night-time and produce melatonin at the right time.

Without these very visible cues of 'daytime equals awake' and 'night-time equals sleep', we not only don't produce the right levels of melatonin, we can also produce other hormones at the wrong time, again making it more challenging to fall asleep. That feeling of pushing through tiredness can result in a second wind, or even a third or fourth wind, meaning streams of adrenaline and cortisol can party through our system, keeping us awake when we want to sleep.

There are practical ways to get a great night's sleep in winter and we can start the preparations in autumn. Something as simple as a daylight lamp during the day can help us feel more alert, and it can also be used to create an artificial sunset at bedtime to induce a natural sleepiness. Straightforward changes can easily be put in place, and we only need to think about these for a few months of the year. Seeing small adjustments as part of our winter plan can set us up for a fantastic night's sleep and give us the energy recharge that we've been seeking.

Sleep hygiene

Sleep hygiene is the slightly strange name for the basic principles of good sleep, which have nothing to do with cleanliness and everything to do with the practices that support us to get a good night's slumber.

A core principle of sleep hygiene is consistency. Going to bed and rising at roughly the same time is key to maintaining a good sleep schedule. Consistency allows your body and brain to create a natural rhythm to your day, which can prepare you for a good night's sleep. If you are constantly varying your sleep schedule, your brain doesn't know when you want to go to sleep and when you want to stay awake.

Although it is not helpful to vary your sleep schedule night by night, it should be varied season by season to align us with nature's rhythms. Overall, a good minimum winter sleep adjustment to make is an additional hour.[9] As already mentioned, very few of us can vary our wake-up time dictated by the alarm clock rousing us for commitments outside of our control. The option we are left with is to go to bed earlier. See this extra sleep as a gift, and remember you only have to embrace it for a season. Focus on what you are prioritizing, such as your health and happiness, not what you are depriving yourself of, such as another hour of TV or social media. This minor adjustment is a necessary adaptation that will make your winter and your life easier, especially if you've been battling lower energy levels. If you struggle with the idea of going to bed or feeling sleepy earlier, then try going to bed just 15 minutes earlier. Once settled into that routine, bring your bedtime forward another 15 minutes, and so on, until you gain your extra hour. This seasonal sleep shift helps you to cope better in winter but also supports you to recuperate from the previous higher-energy seasons.

Be mindful of what your bedroom is for

Ideally, the only activities taking place in your bedroom are sleep and sex. There is significant research showing reading in bed also helps us to sleep, so we can add that to the list, but these should be the *only* activities we do in our bedrooms, and not just at night-time.

When it's cold and grey, many of us can be tempted to stay in the warmth of our bed and pull the laptop onto our lap to work, watch a film, do the online food shop or reply to emails. However, this is a guaranteed way to disrupt our sleep.

Our brains need physical cues for everything. They need a cue that says, 'This is sleep time,' 'This is work time,' 'This is relaxation time,' etc. If we try to make our bedrooms multi-purpose rooms, then our brains won't understand what we are asking of them. If we work from our beds all day, then try to switch off and go to sleep at night, our brains don't recognize that there has been a change. This is particularly true if our tasks look similar. For example, if we are on a laptop and work phone all day, then scroll our phones whilst watching Netflix at night, then all our brains know is that we're looking at a phone and a screen. This means that whilst we are trying to relax and unwind from our working day, our brains are still pushing work thoughts, ideas and problems to the forefront, ruining our enjoyment of the latest boxset. Our brains aren't doing this to annoy us. To be fair to our brains, we are doing the same activities, and there has been no physical cue to switch into 'home' mode, and certainly not into sleep mode. So, no matter how tempting, try to resist doing anything other than sex, sleep and reading in bed, and you are guaranteed a better night's sleep.

Dim the lights

We have to be a little bit more mindful of our surroundings and environment in winter, and in particular pay attention to light. Given that we won't go to bed as soon as it gets dark (around 4pm in the UK in winter), we can spend the majority of our afternoons and evenings under unchanging artificial light. This isn't great for helping us wind down and prepare for a blissful night's slumber. When we switch off an overhead light at bedtime, there has been no wind-down, no gentle fade, no sunset to support our circadian rhythm. Throw some screen and blue-light exposure into the mix, and suddenly you are looking at an environment designed to keep you fully awake, just before bed.

Winter night-time rituals can all be part of winter's soporific gifts. Dim your lights throughout the evening, including your screens. As soon as it gets dark, activate night-time mode on your electronics, such as your phone, tablet, laptop and TV. If you worry that you'll forget to do this, there are apps that change the brightness of your screen according to the time of day and automatically apply night mode to your devices. Alternatively, having them permanently in night mode is no bad thing; it acts as a blue light filter, which minimizes the impact on our melatonin production.

As well as adjusting your screens, try gently dimming the lights around you. If you are watching TV in the evening, turn down the screen brightness, turn off overhead lights and replace them with soft lamps or candlelight. This means you still have plenty of light to see and go about your business, but you are slowly reducing the amount of light you are exposed to.

If reading in bed, try to avoid harsh light. Use a reading lamp or, even better, a bedside sunset lamp, which will gradually dim as you read. Reading is proven to be beneficial for your mental health, with just 30 minutes being shown to lower blood pressure, heart rate and psychological distress.[10] Reading with the right light can be a beautiful winter habit to develop and nurture.

Create a winter bed

There is an energy to our beds and our bedrooms. We feel the palpable difference between a room with an abandoned, crumpled ball of a duvet and one with a freshly made bed.

Clean sheet night is one of those joys in life where the vast pleasure derived completely outweighs the effort required. This weekly act makes me genuinely happy, and the sense of joy from getting under the covers and feeling freshly laundered fabric against my skin is blissful.

I've always liked the energy of clean sheets. I put fresh bed linen on whenever I need an energetic shift. If I have been poorly or developed bed-dread (that feeling where you don't want to go to bed because you are worried you are not going to sleep well), then I imagine washing all that away and starting again with fresh sheets on the bed. A clean slate. A (literal) fresh start.

There are physical changes to my bed in different seasons. I have a heavier and thicker winter duvet, which is perfect for snuggling under when it is chilly. I also have a woollen throw, which adds another layer of welcoming warmth and feels strangely caveman-esque with its weight reminiscent of sleeping under heavy furs.

How do you want *your* bedroom to feel in winter? It's easy to collapse into bed, kicking off clothes, strewing them around the room, leaving the day's detritus in our wake. But our bedroom is the hub of our energy. It is where we start and end our day. It sets us up for the day ahead and completes the journey of another 24 hours. Spending time creating your perfect winter sleeping space will set you up for the season.

What to do when you can't sleep

Have you ever noticed that a problem at 3am feels so much worse than a problem at 3pm? Our brains are not designed to think clearly in the dark. They are designed to scan for threats and consider what action to take to keep us alive. This is an incredibly useful but not very reassuring quirk. It is why we can worry away at a problem in the darkest hours but not come to any solution. Often, a problem can feel very overwhelming and all-consuming in the middle of the night, but our sense of perspective rises with the sun. Once we have daylight, we have clarity. We are not supposed to be problem-solving in the dark, and this can make autumn and winter challenging seasons to get through.

So, what if we don't try to solve problems? What if we accept that we can't make good decisions in the middle of the night and tell ourselves we will address the problem again during daylight hours? What happens if we simply sit in the dark with winter?

> *It's 3am and I've been awake since 2.30am. I try not to clock-watch because it interferes with sleep,*[11] *but the consistent and unvarying darkness of a winter night makes it harder to place myself in my sleep cycle. If it's 10 minutes before my alarm goes off, then I'll stay awake; if I have hours left to go, then I will try to go back to sleep, but even as I check the time, I already know it's not happening. I am fully awake. I creep out of the bedroom and hear the gentle thud-thud as both dogs sleepily jump off their bed to follow me downstairs to see what I am up to. The eldest sits by my feet to supervise the making of hot chocolate. I open the fridge, closing my eyes against the light and reaching with the sight of habit for the milk. I take my mug over to the small squashy sofa at the back of our kitchen, where the pup has already stretched out, claiming her spot in anticipation. As I sit, after a*

bit of negotiating and gentle hip bumping with the dogs, I find myself gazing through the patio doors, utterly captivated by the full effulgence of the brightest moon I've ever seen. It is so beautiful that I want to undo all my considerate creeping and padding around and run upstairs to shake my partner awake so he can see this. Equally, so transfixed am I, that I am reluctant to miss a single second. Sure enough, mere moments later, the plenilune is hidden by a wisp of cloud. I now know that this is why I was awake. My head had been spinning, and winter wanted to show me that even in the darkest moments, there is brightness. There is beauty. I pull a throw around me and find my thoughts drifting, yet I make no attempt to catch them. I stay here for about 40 minutes, cuddling my snoring dogs, cradling my cuppa and looking out at the sky. I feel nothing but a deep-seated peace. Despite it necessitating a lack of sleep, I want this feeling again. I don't feel isolated or cross or worried about how I will cope later that day. I know I will. I know that this moment, sitting with winter, is restoring me, not depleting me, and I feel totally at ease.

Being with winter in the darkest hours

1. Set yourself up with a cosy corner
If you share a bedroom, then sitting up in bed, putting the lamp on and reaching for your current book could be deemed anti-social in the wee hours. It's also not in keeping with the hours

that I am talking about here. It's not about being productive. It's not about 'making use' of the time. It's about being in winter, with winter, sitting together contemplating the night sky.

A cosy corner is somewhere you can retreat to in the dark; it may even be your winter retreat spot. Wherever it is, make sure that it's somewhere you can escape to undisturbed.

2. Keep warm

The night chill can be off-putting in winter, as the house temperature often plummets, so you want to keep your warmest, snuggliest clothes nearby to envelop the heat of your slumber and carry it with you to your cosy corner. I have a huge fluffy dressing gown that I love (despite my inherent resemblance to the cookie monster when wearing it), and I have the advantage of two cockapoos who are only too willing to act as hot-water bottles in exchange for a bit of fuss. Have something nearby that you can cocoon into with minimal effort to keep warm and cosy.

3. Have a no-plan plan

When I get up in the middle of the night and head downstairs, the temptation to 'do' something is overwhelming. My brain rushes with thoughts of 'I'll just stack the dishwasher,' 'I could put a wash on, and it'll be ready by the time we're up for work,' 'I have been meaning to scan my receipts for my tax return . . .' etc. Don't be pulled in. This is not a punishing early-morning wake-up call to cram yet more into your day. This is an invitation from winter to spend some of your calmest moments simply being, without expectation or output. My personal plan usually involves a hot drink because I need no encouragement to grab a hot chocolate, and I love cradling the mug and stealing some warmth. Create a plan of what you are going to do in that quiet time with winter, and make sure it's a no-plan plan.

4. Do not disturb

My other half is well used to what he calls my wombling, and so knows there is no requirement to follow me downstairs and enquire about my health. In fact, he knows that this time is time for me and that I will come back to bed, revelling in the warmth, having cooled down outside of the covers, and snuggle in when I am ready and I feel sleepy once more. I think this is important. I have had partners in the past abruptly flick light switches on and demand, 'What are you doing?' and it made me jump, shattering the peace that had settled as I sat quietly. Make sure that those around you know that nothing is wrong, they don't need to do anything, you are simply spending some moments with winter.

5. Arrange your day ahead

Given we find it more difficult to problem-solve in the dark, there is an argument for arranging our day and our activities to align with daylight as much as possible. If we have heavier cognitive work to complete, or we need to solve something challenging, then we are better to rearrange our diary to accommodate that in the brightest part of the day. If we have broken sleep or troubled sleep, then rearranging our day so we are doing our hardest work with the most resources supporting us makes sense. It is a small winter adjustment, but being mindful of our energy and thought patterns in winter can be the difference between feeling productive or thwarted.

6. Know that you are not alone

If ever you are looking at the moon, you are definitely not alone. When my partner and I used to live apart, looking at the same moon was one of the ways that we stayed connected, even when we couldn't physically be in the same place. When you are looking at the moon, so are countless others. We are a middle-of-the-night community, and so if ever you feel isolated or lonely, then look at the moon and feel the golden thread of gentle connection linking you with hundreds of thousands of others.

Accepting a winter sleep

Winter is a time for gentleness. For adjusting. A reshifting of energy and focus. 'Pushing through' in winter serves no one and the same applies to your sleep habits. I encourage you to scan your energy levels and check in to see how you feel. We need to be mindful of what we are sleeping to recover from. As Dallas Hartwig writes in his book *The 4 Season Solution*, 'We industrialized humans burn the metaphorical candle at both ends . . . with a blowtorch.'[12] If we lived in off-grid cabins and walked all day, breathing fresh mountain air, never worrying about Wi-Fi or Zoom meetings, then pushing through with a few short hours of sleep may be enough for us to rise and feel energized and focused. But throw into the mix the storm that is modern living, and suddenly the ratio of brain rest to brain activity is woefully inadequate. The reality for most of us is that we will benefit from more sleep, and winter provides the perfect setting to achieve this. Winter sleep offers the foundational fertile ground in which we plant our hopes, dreams, plans and goals for the year ahead.

The quieter, gentler, softer hush of our winter sleep can continue as we languidly stretch into our day. Step softly into today. What is winter offering you? How can you embrace it?

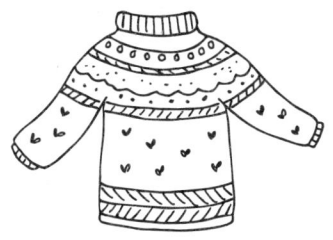

Chapter 7:
The fabric of winter

Like a moth to a flame, I am drawn to winter clothes. The second the stores start stocking their winter wares, I cannot resist. I am incapable of walking past without stopping to lovingly stroke a sleeve. There is something so comforting and alluring in the soft and fluffy textures on offer. There is warmth and pleasure woven into the luxurious fabrics: velvety scarves, merino wool jumpers, cashmere blends. But this isn't about price, it's about feel, and enticing textures are everywhere in winter. I feel an instinctive pull, as though these clothes are calling to me. I simply have to touch them.

My obsession with softness is not unique to me. Our hands and fingertips are amazingly sensitive to texture. When we come into contact with an object or surface, information is transmitted from sensors in the skin, through the nerves, to the somatosensory cortex, which is the part of the brain responsible for interpreting our sense of touch.

Research shows that neurons in this part of the brain will

respond differently to different surfaces as they process what we touch.[1] Whilst we can easily distinguish between coarse sandpaper and smooth glass, we can also detect more subtle differences across a wide range of textures, such as the sheen of silk or the soft give of cotton.[2] Some neurons will react to the roughness or spatial pattern of a texture, others will respond to finer details, certain patterns of indentations in the skin that occur with touch. This is how we know if our bedsheets have a high or low thread count without looking. The variety in the response of our neurons and receptors allows for the richness of the sensation we feel.[3] It is our subtle-feature-detecting neurons that allow us to fall completely in love with our winter wardrobes.

Fabrics have the ability to make us feel happy, safe and secure. Our brains catalogue the feel, weight and shape of everything we've ever touched and store this information in our haptic memory. When all this knowledge is stored in our brains, it is intertwined with other sensory or emotional memories, meaning we remember how an object or texture made us feel, as well as the feel of the object or texture itself.[4]

The multisensory encoding of memory in this way offers us a far superior recollection of an event or object than single-sensory encoding.[5] Simply put, we better retain information when several of our senses are involved in an experience.

If you are someone who prefers the feel of a paperback to reading on your phone or Kindle, then the research is in your corner. We retain the message of a book we have held better than the message of a digital publication because all of our senses are engaged in the process. If we remember a message better when it is printed on paper, and our sensory memories interact, it makes sense that a pleasant texture will create a pleasant memory of what we read. As linguist Naomi Baron explained, 'Smell and sight are relevant senses when it comes to reading, but touch may well be the most important.'[6]

The Japanese concept of *shitsukan* explains how the sensory characteristics of materials affect how we perceive them. Our brains will use the sensory information and attribute qualities to the material. For example, the weight of an object will affect how desirable that object is to us. When presented with a heavy menu, we will consider the food to be of a higher standard than when presented with a lighter menu.[7] Textures that have a high level of friction (think cling film) are more likely to be disliked.[8] Advertisements printed on premium paper create a perception of uniqueness and exclusivity.[9] Textures considered subjectively softer are preferred to those considered rougher.[10] What we touch and how we interpret the texture matters and can change how we feel about an object. Also, the language we use to describe textures and emotions are intertwined. It is possible to have a 'rough week'. We can describe a process as being 'as smooth as silk'. Our innermost feelings influence how we experience textures and vice versa.[11] Smooth and soft textures elicit positive emotions, whilst rough and coarse textures elicit negative ones.

This explains our lust for all things soft, cosy, snuggly and reassuring in texture. Soft fabrics provide a barrier against the harshness of the world, which feels especially important in winter when the temperatures invite us to cocoon. If you're having a bad day, I encourage you to dress in textures that offer a comforting hug and ignite a spark of happiness within you.

> 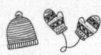 **Activity: Connecting with a softer winter**
>
> Take a moment to run your hands over your winter clothes. Take your time, close your eyes and focus on the feel, give and pull of each fabric and the emotions they elicit in you. How do the textures of your clothes make you feel? Now consider how you *want* to feel in winter and how you can use the textures of your wardrobe to achieve that feeling. If you want winter to feel softer, cosier, gentler and more comfortable, then make sure that these are the textures around you. Select the outfit that offers you the biggest hug of softness and move it to the very front of your wardrobe, ready to embrace you when you need it the most.

Dressing for winter

Alfred Wainwright wrote in his 1973 book *A Coast to Coast Walk* that there is no such thing as bad weather, just unsuitable clothing, and I wholeheartedly agree with him.[12] The only time I dislike the weather, at any time of year, is when I am not dressed for it. There is immense satisfaction in getting it right. If I step out in the rain wearing my long waterproof jacket and wellies, then I am completely covered and arrive home bone-dry. I have no issue with the weather in winter *as long as I am dressed for it*.

There is no denying that winter is cold. If we're not a fan of cooler temperatures, the seasonal chill can be challenging. My colleague Priya once told me that her summer and winter work wardrobes were exactly the same. Priya's rationale was that she had a short tube ride to work and then sat in a temperature-controlled office, so she didn't see the point in having different wardrobes for different seasons. Although Priya always looked infinitely glamorous, I couldn't understand why she didn't make any adjustments through the seasons, especially as she *hated* winter and constantly complained of feeling cold.

Similarly, I follow a fashion influencer on Instagram and truly love her work. Yet, year-on-year, her posts have become repetitive complaints about the weather. Said influencer loves the sunshine, and anything else causes a daily (sometimes hourly) moan to her followers. Given she is UK-based, you can imagine there is a lot of reason for moaning! Whilst I wouldn't dream of offering a fashion guru advice on what to wear, if I knew her better, I would be compelled to point out that the weather is not the problem; her wardrobe is. This influencer openly discusses how she doesn't wear socks; she steps outside in February in leather-look leggings with nothing but a thong underneath, and the only warm accessory is her smile. No wonder this fashionista doesn't like the weather. She doesn't dress for it. Neither does Priya. It's hard to feel any warmth towards winter when we are shivering, stylistically stuck in summer.

Many people don't buy winter clothes because to do so is to admit defeat and concede that they are indeed having to face winter. This reminds me of revenge bedtime procrastination with its sense of cutting your nose off to spite your face, and it serves us just as well. We can struggle uncomfortably through the changing seasons, only relaxing when we arrive at the one that suits our wardrobe, but there is a reality to plummeting temperatures. If you're already not a fan of winter, you may resent spending money on the appropriate clothes, but not doing so makes the season infinitely harder. If we are layering, then our winter wardrobe can be used throughout the year, meaning any investment stretches a lot further than a one-off summery dress. All the gorgeous caresses that wait in warm, cuddlesome clothes are wasted unless you invest in winter – and it doesn't need to bust the budget.

In true 'commercialism doesn't support us' style, the best time to buy winter clothes is . . . in the summer. When everyone is googling 'Are air conditioner units worth it?' it is the perfect time to begin searching for your winter wardrobe. Summer shopping for winter clothing allows us to realistically budget for what we might need. One year, my partner bought a coat worth £189, and it cost him £40. We blinked at the label, then took it to the till, where the chap laughed at our confusion and said, 'I know, right? Unbelievable, but yes, you're reading it right.' Just £40 for a high-quality, double-layer, fleece-lined raincoat that will last him for years. When did we buy this item? In one of the hottest weeks on record at the end of June.

It's a bizarre mind-shift to make, for sure, but once you have your list of winter wants, it's easy enough to periodically search for these throughout the year. Think of this shopping as part of the season's preparations. You buy suncream, sunnies and sandals for summer. You need wellies, waterproofs and warmth for winter.

There are many budget-friendly and sustainable options. Charity shops and second-hand auction sites often provide a great source of winter wares, especially for children, as they rapidly grow out of seasonal clothes, meaning you can pick up something near-new for very little.

You don't have to spend a fortune, but you do need to see your winter wardrobe as worthy of *some* investment. Just as in cold countries you have to budget for winter tyres, budgeting for winter clothes will keep you feeling happier, safer, snuggly and more secure. Moreover, this will help you to attain previously unfelt levels of satisfaction when the weather turns, but you are appropriately dressed and remain unfazed. Keeping your winter wardrobe in mind allows you to buy clothes that will last you for years and that will return season after season to hug you, warm you and comfort you.

When did winter get so grey?

Our lives have become a little greyer over the last decade or so. I'm not talking about depressing global events (although, obvs) but rather speaking literally about the increased love of grey as a colour. Both in and out of our homes, grey seems to have taken over as *the* colour of choice.

My lovely friend Jane's husband once grumbled to me, 'If Jane had her way, the inside of our home would resemble a battleship.' When my partner and I moved into our home, the previous owners had such a love of the colour that every room was painted a slightly varying dark shade of grey. It was like living in a cave.

European homes have also seen the rise of simple, plain, clean lines, often referred to as a Nordic or Scandi look, which was closely followed by a trend for minimalism. Combine these looks with the current grey overtone, and what you are left with is grey and . . . little else.

Colour really matters. I am not a big shopper, but I do love seeing all the summer colours adorning mannequins in the shop windows. I love walking around and seeing people wearing hot pink and floral patterns. There is a fantastic statement in summer clothing; it says vibrancy, freshness and boldness. There is something wonderful about the zest of lime green or burnt orange. These are colours to dance in, jump in, do anything other than stay still in. The fabrics come to life as they float and swirl, energetically moving with our bodies. The weather may not always play ball, but the textures and colours of summer invite playfulness, laughter and joy.

Autumn and winter clothes tell a different story. Right in the middle of this cascade of colour, along comes something sensible, heavy and dark to ruin the vibe. I've never really understood why the clothes that we are sold for winter are black, brown or grey. I don't understand why, when the weather is at its dullest, we enter into a dullness competition along with it. It is almost as though we are being told, 'Don't enjoy winter, it's not for joy. Winter is a time for dark, depressing blackness. The fun stops here. It's time to leave the party. Put your (dull) coat on.'

Research tells us that the colours we surround ourselves with have a big impact on our mood.[13] Red is associated with strong emotions such as love and passion. Orange is associated with excitement; yellow with cheerfulness and joy; green with nature and money; blue with loyalty, honesty and reliability; and purple with creativity, mystery and royalty.

The research on black, brown and grey paints a very different picture. In one study, 51% of respondents associated black with sadness.[14] Grey affects the mind and body by causing unsettling feelings. Too much grey not only creates feelings of sadness and depression, it also evokes feelings of loneliness and isolation.[15] Brown, another dark colour, can also evoke feelings of loneliness, sadness and further isolation.[16] The colours we surround ourselves with will affect everything from our mood, concentration and motivation through to our confidence and friendliness.¹⁷ Our envelopment in the darker end of the colour spectrum during winter goes some way to explain why we may also be enveloped in a darker mood.

Essentially, the winter wardrobe staples of brown, black and grey could contribute to feelings of depression, loneliness and isolation. Perhaps it isn't the season itself that makes us feel this way, but the way we dress for it. Who decided that winter needs to be drab? If we are dressing that way, then no wonder we feel down and sad. Winter is the perfect time to add colour, to cheer not just you but everyone around you. You can be a literal ray of sunshine in amongst the gloomy crowd. My winter wardrobe is full of royal blue, emerald green, hot pink, burnt orange and sunflower yellow. In fact, my wardrobe is more colourful in winter than at any other time of the year, and I'd encourage you to follow suit. When we mute our colours, we mute our mood.

As a student, I had a coat in bright royal blue with a hot pink lining, and it was magnificent. Stepping out in my coat, I felt as though the rest of the world had been edited to monochrome whilst my coat was highlighted in colour. I felt happy, bright, vibrant and bold. Strangers smiled at me more. Despite the unspoken agreement of non-communication we all seem to adhere to on public transport, people broke the silence just to tell me that they loved my coat. My colourful coat also hid a multitude of sartorial sins; if I looked a bit scruffy or hastily put together, then my coat did some serious heavy lifting in the glamour stakes. But more importantly, that coat gave me a daily mood boost, and I've never looked back, slipping colour into my winter wardrobe wherever I can. My umbrella is a giant sunflower. My nails are bright coral or jewel red, deliberately chosen because, as a writer, I see my hands a lot. I try to wear colour in every outfit, every day, and I feel better as a result.

I appreciate not everyone wants to dress in sunshine yellow, but it doesn't need to be over the top to be impactful. In winter, we have so many more options because, typically, we are wearing more than one layer, so we can add colour with a scarf, a bag or a pair of socks. Give yourself an uplift in mood by weaving more vibrancy through your garments, and see how it makes you feel.

We are surrounded by natural colour in winter with red berries, yellow leaves, green buds and inky blue skies. The colours we choose can mirror nature's colour palette and the inspiriting energy around us that glitters with shimmering frosts. It takes as much effort to put on a colourful outfit as a dull one, but our mood will thank us for the colourful upgrade. What is one splash of colour that you could add to your outfit today? How does it make you feel?

The effortless glamour of winter

I've always viewed winter as a very glamorous season. I used to see women in magazines wearing the softest cashmere, playfully pulling sleeves down over manicured nails, donning a jaunty hat or an enveloping scarf, and I wanted to be like them.

There is something very easy about dressing in winter. I tend to live in a uniform of jeans with a soft, colourful jumper, and it's a fairly effortless look. Throw on some jewellery and a bit of make-up, and suddenly you look ready for a pub lunch or a night out in a way that you just don't in summer.

With half-English and half-Irish heritage, my skin could be described as 'English rose' if you were being kind, or 'astonishingly pale' if you were being honest. Perhaps if I wasn't so pale, or I had better tolerance to the sun (I have the kind of skin tone that looks as though it would burn under a 60W bulb), I'd feel differently. But when it comes to my wardrobe, I feel much more oppressed in summer.

Whilst the films may show us bronzed legs escaping from silky wisps of barely there dresses, my personal experience of summer sees me red, hot and bothered. I am permanently trying to balance a cold drink, along with every other item I need to have to hand because no summer clothing seems to have pockets. Summer sees me trying to discreetly glance at my underarms to check for sweat patches or sniffing for scented evidence of the same. This doesn't scream glamour to me.

By contrast, my winter wardrobe of jeans, jumpers, fluffy cardigans, boots and scarves makes me feel put together and confident. Everything feels beautiful and elegant, and I cannot get enough. I genuinely adore winter dressing. Spending time wrapped in snuggly, cosy layers of delectable softness feels as though I am having a continual hug from my wardrobe. It's an embrace I welcome every year.

A winter wardrobe audit

When faced with the dull palette of traditional winter staples (brown, black, grey), it's too easy to grab the nearest, cleanest or warmest item of clothing and think, 'That'll do,' but this isn't going to inspire you to have your best day or experience your best mood. We can all be guilty of pulling on the same misshapen fleece four days in a row and then wondering why we feel less than motivated. This is not about seeking external validation. We should all dress in a way that works for us. This is about *you* and the impact your clothes have on you.

A little forward planning can help you to feel not just prepared but amazing. It is disheartening to pull a jumper on over a shirt, only to realize that the collar doesn't sit comfortably and that you are going to be awkwardly readjusting all day. Similarly, if you want to wear that cute dress over thick black tights with boots, only to remember that your last pair of tights fell victim to the cat's claws and that your boots are scuffed and looking less than loved, then you can find yourself feeling less willing to face the day.

It isn't silly or frivolous to dedicate time to our wardrobe. What we wear will dictate everything from how sociable we feel and how much interaction we will have, right the way through to the emotions we are primed to experience. Your clothes matter, not for other people's approval but for your own sense of self.

Activity: Winter wardrobe audit

Put some time aside when you won't be distracted and gather up every item of winter clothing. I don't just mean your big coat; I mean your jumpers, shoes, trainers, boots, jeans, jackets and wellies. Anything you wear in winter, add to the pile. Next, following the famous Marie Kondo approach, consider each item carefully and ask, 'Does this spark joy for me?' Then consider whether it still fits you. How do you feel when you wear it? What weather is this item best suited to? The weather factor is important to consider, as some jumpers are amazingly snuggly indoors but absolutely useless if it's blowing a gale because they let the wind whistle through and chill you to the bone.

Once you have a pile of winter clothes that fit well and spark joy, ask yourself what gaps there are in your wardrobe. Where do you need to restock or rebuy? What can you look out for in the sales and auction sites? Make a list and keep it with you, so you have it to hand whenever you are out shopping or scrolling. Minimum effort but maximum result.

Next, gather your outfits together. I recommend having a handful of go-to looks that you feel amazing in and hanging them as complete outfits in your wardrobe. Include your accessories and keep the right shoes directly underneath. Then, when you open your wardrobe in the morning, you are greeted with a selection of outfits that you know make you feel good. (Bonus points for saving yourself from decision fatigue before your day has begun – more on that in the next chapter).

Like all aspects of winter, these simple adjustments and adaptations can help make the season easier for us. Embrace the fabrics of winter, and they will embrace you right back.

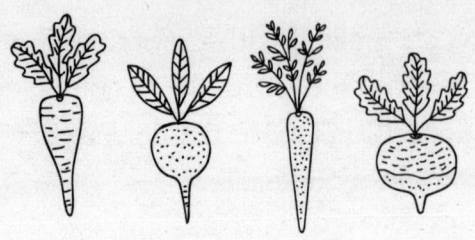

Chapter 8:
The taste of winter

There is a taste to winter. Particular foods carry the scents, flavours and memories of the season, and much of the warmth of winter's embrace comes from what we eat and drink. We rarely crave a stick of celery straight from the fridge on an icy, cold day. The foods we want to eat are those that warm us from the inside out, an edible central heating system. Asking a friend what she wanted for dinner, she replied, 'Something hearty, something warming . . . you know, something wintery.' I knew exactly what she meant. Winter food is soul food and nourishes us from head to toe whilst warming our hearts.

Much of the food we eat in winter comes from the ground; it is a literal connection with the earth and nature around us. Whereas summer food grows on trees or vines, high off the ground and basking in the sunshine, winter food is earthier. These seasonal foods reflect the energetic shift in nature. Sun-kissed vine fruits are a living metaphor for higher summer energy and altitude. Having absorbed goodness and nutrients from the earth it grew in, winter produce offers a reconnection to fuel our bodies and reunite us with nature.

The tastes of winter are deep and sophisticated, comprising flavours and spices which cause our tastebuds to dance. Although powerful in flavour, winter food is gentle in pace. Slowly reducing stews. One-pot dishes. Roast dinners. These all take time, and the flavours mature and evolve throughout the cooking process. What a beautiful example of winter energy. A palatable encouragement to ease the rush. Not only that, but these foods take longer to eat. Whereas a sandwich can be eaten in moments, a hot meal takes time to cool, and we must wait before we can enjoy it. These pauses at mealtimes are invitations: they are a time for us, a time to relax, a time to talk, a time to recharge our batteries after a busy day. Rather than a grab-and-go dining option, winter food offers a mealtime retreat.

For me, being cooked for is one of the greatest gifts. It doesn't need to be anything extravagant; even the heating up of a ready meal means the world because it's not about the food itself, it's about the effort someone else has put into ensuring I am fed. With the average adult making around 35,000 decisions per day,[1] by the time dinner rolls around, we are mentally spent. Even though many of our decisions are automatic, made using subconsciously stored information, many others require active thought and consideration, and these build up and take their toll. Decision fatigue is very real, and at the end of the day, we are less likely to be able to make clear decisions, even if it's something seemingly as small as what to eat. To have someone else take control and relieve me of one further decision makes me want to weep with gratitude.

The other benefit of being cooked for is eating together. Communal eating increases our wellbeing and sense of social bonding, as well as making us feel connected with our community.[2] That said, eating together is not always easy. The average adult eats 10 meals out of 21 alone every week,[3] mainly due to hectic schedules and clashing priorities, making it difficult to come together and eat with friends and family.

Even living with others doesn't mean we eat together: 21% of adults say clashes in evening routines mean that they eat at different times to others in their household. Of those who do eat together, less than half sit together at the kitchen table.[4] This is true across age ranges and occurs for many reasons, including different dietary requirements and who we live with (families and flatmates are unlikely to share dining habits). However, our modern-day distractions also create a barrier to connection, with two-thirds of us engaging in distracted dining, watching either the television or another screen or device whilst we eat.

Paying attention to what we eat is good for us, both for our bodies and our brains. Mindful eating is not about focusing on *what* we eat so much as *how* we eat. It's tuning into our emotional state, our feelings of hunger and fullness. When we are distracted, we are much more likely to overeat, as we miss our internal cues that tell us we are feeling full.[5] This leads us to experience significant digestive discomfort, which can then prevent us from sleeping well. We are also likely to continue over-eating because we have a less distinct memory of our food intake. Meals that are eaten in a distracted state have been shown to be less satisfying. We enjoy our food less when we are in front of a screen, which means we eat more, as we seek the satisfaction of the food that we busily ignored when our attention was elsewhere.

There is a powerful emotional connection with our food. Being aware of our emotional state as we eat is important. It allows us to tune into our choices and how they support our overall wellbeing. When we are busy and distracted, it is hard to listen to our bodies and uncover what we need. This digestive disconnect doesn't serve us well, reducing our enjoyment of food and creating negative associations.

We build memories through food, with different scents and flavours transporting us back to a different time. The hippocampus has strong links to the parts of the brain connected to emotional memories and smell, which is why the scent of freshly brewed coffee takes me back to being a child standing in my grandparents' kitchen. The hippocampus directly links to our digestive system through its role in processing food cues, regulating appetite and forming memories related to eating. Many hormones that regulate our appetite, digestion and behaviour have receptors in the hippocampus, meaning food is something around which memories are formed. Our brains are primed to pay attention to food, and when we are fully present during meals with others, we can form strong bonds and strong memories.

Winter offers us the opportunity to sit and eat together, sharing stories in the pauses as our food cools and we prepare to eat. We can create memories, laughter and joy through the food we share, and on a very practical note, winter dishes are often the most budget-friendly of the year. Seasonal root and cruciferous vegetables are readily and cheaply available and make for filling and nourishing stews and soups. Winter is a great time to host others at your table, but even if you don't want to cook, you can arrange a meal with friends or family. Perhaps everyone brings a dish, or you meet at a favourite café or restaurant. The setup is not important but the attention and community around our food is, allowing us to enjoy the memories we cook up together.

A disconnected diet

International food imports mean that we can now eat whatever we want at any time of year. Strawberries in December? Sure. Smashed avocado on toast all year round? Why not. Indeed, our own attitudes towards sustainability and increasing awareness of the impact of food miles are the only real inhibitors of what we put on our plates. Our diets, like so much else, are out of sync with the natural world. We would be hard-pushed to deduce the season from the wares displayed in the supermarket or on our dining tables. Our food showcases preference and habit, not the season.

Research evaluating the choices of thousands of French and US participants found that people repeatedly ate the same meal for breakfast.[6] Although they sought variety for lunch and dinner, breakfast was the one meal that people were happy to repeat, day in, day out, throughout the week. We know what we like and we know what fits with our morning routine, and we rarely alter it.

Breakfast is an indicator to start our day; a comestible cue for our brains that it is morning now and we need to prepare for our day ahead. We rarely alter our diets to reflect a more seasonal start to the day. Whilst breakfast may be a meal that we are reluctant to change, hosting winter at our dining tables does have huge physical and mental health benefits, and it is worth looking at where touches of winter can be added to your daily menu.

Prior to the modern world's transportation, refrigeration and other food miracles, our diets would have reflected the seasons around us. Our tastes and desires would have aligned with nature, our cravings curbed by scarcity of ingredients. Our brains have developed over time to crave and thrive on the foods of the season to ensure nourishment and nutrients. Winter offers us what we need through seasonal winter crops but it's easy to ignore this when we can have literally anything we want.

Our seasonal rhythm mismatch means we work against our bodies and what they need. Our bodies crave protein and root vegetables in winter. This craving has been formed by hundreds of years of what was available. It's also a noticeably lean diet. Yet I've had many conversations with friends where they (and I) will bemoan what we deem to be the inevitable winter weight gain. If our brains desire a lean, healthy diet of protein and vegetables, why do we believe we will put weight on?

Quite simply, because we do. Our mindset matters, and if we expect to put weight on, we probably will. There is an accepted popular myth that we will put on around 5lbs over the winter months, and this is presented with inevitability. It's just what happens. We *will* get a bit heavier over winter. Many of us see the festive season as a period of indulgence and January is saddled with the resulting penance (which could be another reason why we take a dislike to the start of winter, as we associate it with deprivation and lack).

We allow ourselves to gain a few pounds by indulging in more alcohol, more mince pies, more snacks, more party food. We may allow ourselves to eat without restriction in December because . . . well . . . Christmas! Although, in my eyes, winter weight gain doesn't matter a jot in terms of aesthetics, we need to pay attention to what we are eating and how it is supporting our overall wellbeing. The phrase 'listen to your body' is all too often met with an eye-roll, but it is the simplest feedback loop we have. Eat, tune in, listen. Do we feel good or bad after the food we've eaten? There's our feedback, and that feedback is a gift.

Before I knew I had SAD, when I felt low and emotional, junk foods provided a source of succour. It's called comfort eating for a reason and though I really embraced it, it didn't love me back. Foods that are nutritionally empty often leave us feeling empty too. The plethora of junk food thrown at us all through 'party season' can make us feel painfully bloated but also still hungry. Although we are eating (often overeating), we rarely feel full or satisfied.

When we are in the season of rest and recuperation, we need to listen to what our bodies are asking for. When I tuned in to what my body needed in winter and ate accordingly, I realized I was eating seasonally. It turned out that everything my body was asking for was readily available to me. No air miles or avocadoes in sight. Winter provided me with hearty, wholesome, beautiful food which nourished my body and boosted my mood. I didn't need to import expensive ingredients or stomp a heavy carbon footprint on our planet. Inviting winter to my table proved cheaper, more sustainable and more supportive of my overall health and wellbeing, and it's something we can all benefit from.

The taste of winter is flavoured and nuanced, and there is a little magic in winter cooking, which lies in the healing and restorative properties of warming winter spices.

Kitchen magic

A few years ago, I was packed onto a rush-hour tube carriage with hundreds of harassed commuters keen to make connections at London Paddington. As the doors opened and people surged forward, I was unceremoniously pushed out of the train and landed awkwardly on my ankle. Being British and therefore mortified at the notion of (whisper it) making a fuss, I ignored the white-hot jolt of pain that shot through me and ran for my train. As I watched my ankle swell with alarming rapidity, I knew I was in real trouble. The train crew kindly helped me off the train at my stop, and I hobbled home. Unbeknownst to me, this wasn't a sprain but the result of a small chip of bone coming away on impact and becoming lodged in my ankle joint. It was as painful as it sounds, if not a smidge more. When extensive physio and ankle manipulation yielded no improvement, I headed into surgery. I returned home with crutches, a rehabilitation programme and some very strong painkillers, which my body unhelpfully rejected. Beyond paracetamol, which didn't touch the sides, I was stuck, and so I turned to food. However, I wasn't comfort eating. I was seeking to soothe and heal.

My kitchen cupboards replaced my medicine cabinet as I researched what I should be eating. Ginger has wonderful anti-nausea and anti-inflammatory properties, and no matter how much I ate or drank, I wanted more. My ankle puffiness lessened along with the pain as I made endless cups of a simple hot ginger tea, grating fresh ginger into a mug and adding boiling water. The punch it packed was powerful, but ginger is such a warming, welcoming hug of a spice that it was also intensely comforting to a body battered by surgery and pain.

Further research highlighted the power of turmeric, which has strong anti-inflammatory properties and complements ginger really well. Working together, they can help alleviate anxiety and depression. I felt remarkably cheered as I sat there drinking my golden milk – a hot turmeric drink which is utterly delicious – and eating my fresh ginger biscuits (I decided it all counts). I then turned my attention to garlic, which has countless medicinal properties. It dawned on me that my core three ingredients – turmeric, garlic and ginger – would make an incredibly flavoursome base for a curry, and so Steph's Super Healing Curry was born.

This dish has become a kitchen staple of mine. Whenever I am feeling poorly, or my body or mind needs to heal, my Super Healing Curry is created. Friends of mine, whether healing a broken bone or a broken heart, get served this dish, and I've had more than one tearful request that has warranted a late-night dash to the shops to procure fresh ginger and chillies to create culinary comfort.

Food is about so much more than just nourishment for me. The innate healing properties of this curry go beyond the ingredients and reside in the intention of the dish. It is made with love. I make it in the hope of making someone feel better, and that hope gets stirred in along with the spices. I want this dish to support, encourage and warm the soul. Feeding someone a dish filled with healing powers and love is a form of care that only really plays out in winter. The seasonal vegetables and fresh flavours are best served wrapped in the comforting dark blanket of a winter night. Tears are mopped with tissues, whilst sauce is mopped with naan bread. I hope that in sharing this recipe, you can cook it for yourself, for your friends, for those in your life who need support and those who you want to hug and heal.

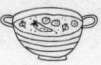 **Steph's Super Healing Curry:**

Serves 2–4 people (depending on hunger levels)
Vegan*

2 tbsp vegetable oil

1 red onion

3 cloves of garlic, crushed

4cm piece of fresh root ginger, finely grated

1 red chilli, deseeded and thinly sliced

1 tbsp ground turmeric

1 tsp ground cumin

1 tsp ground coriander

1 tsp garam masala

1kg sweet potatoes, chopped into medium (2–3cm) chunks. Leave skin on for added flavour and goodness.

2 courgettes, diced into medium chunks (as above)

1 small aubergine, diced into medium chunks (as above)

400ml good-quality vegetable stock

200g baby spinach

a handful of fresh coriander, chopped (including stalks)

freshly ground salt and black pepper, for seasoning

Dried chilli flakes, for serving (if you like a little extra spice)

1) Heat the vegetable oil in a large saucepan or stock pot over a medium heat and add the onion. Cook for 4–5 minutes, then add the garlic, ginger and chillies and cook until softened slightly.
2) Add all the spices and stir through to coat evenly.
3) Add the sweet potato and the vegetable stock, stir, adjust the heat to a gentle simmer, cover with a lid and cook for 10 minutes. Add the courgettes and aubergine and cook for a further 10–15 minutes, or until the sweet potato has softened.
4) Add the spinach and season with salt and pepper to taste.
5) Serve the curry sprinkled with fresh coriander and a smattering of dried chilli flakes, if desired.

I recommend eating with delicious warm naan bread, a bed of hot rice or mixed vegetables (simply steamed and served loaded with the curry – delicious!).

* This recipe is vegan but you could absolutely add chicken or other protein to the mix if you wanted to. If adding meat, add it to the pan after step 2 and cook until browned/sealed. Ensure that the meat is thoroughly cooked before serving. Also throw in any other veg that you fancy. This curry can take a lot of playing with and will easily absorb flavours, so listen to your body and enjoy every bite.

Cooking in winter

My idea of a perfect Sunday is some uninterrupted time in the kitchen. I love nothing more than having the oven on, a podcast playing or some catch-up TV on the iPad whilst I get busy creating. Before writing, none of my jobs ever had a tangible end product. My love of cooking and baking comes from the sense of satisfaction of taking a fully formed loaf out of the oven or being able to offer a slice of homemade cake with a cup of tea at my kitchen table.

Of all the cooking that I do, cooking in winter holds a particularly special place in my heart. Preparing food in summer is more about putting simple ingredients together. I'll throw together a salad, grate white cabbage, carrot and apple for coleslaw, season meat for a barbeque. There is very little actual cooking involved. Summer cooking is assembly, gathering and preparing. I still enjoy it, but it feels rushed. It is delivered with a high-paced energy that is fitting for summer. Like a bee diving for some pollen and then flying away, summer eating is grazing, fast and quick. Whatever lets us get out and get on, so that we can plug back into summer's high-frequency energy.

Winter cooking is something else. It's combining flavours, it's being snugly huddled in the kitchen, sampling spices, adding warmth and nourishment, seeking how to get as many nutrients into a dish as possible. My kitchen becomes a hygge space. I have the radio on, the oven on and the hob on. I am warm and rosy-cheeked, my natural curls escaping attempts at restraint and springing out, encouraged by the steam from lifted pan lids and the blast of warmth that rushes out of the open oven door.

On a practical note, the kitchen is also a wonderful place to stay cosy and warm. It becomes a steamy den filled with a welcoming sense of love. The end result is satisfying, but there's also comfort and escape in the actual process. Cooking can mindfully absorb us, and we feel good for doing it. Research shows that cooking can boost our confidence and self-esteem and result in better mental clarity and focus. The mindfulness of cooking, focusing on one task, is a huge part of the benefit, and we can share it with others. It's not just eating together that connects us; the process and preparation of food can also boost our connection, and it can be a brilliant activity to do with children or friends.

The love of food

I can be transported to my childhood and infinite happy memories of being with my grandparents when I smell my grandmother's bread toasting. I remember the solid form of my dad beating pancake batter with full-body vigour every Shrove Tuesday. I think of my mum every time I make anything with lemons because she loves the fresh citrus flavour. I use food to show my love for people, and I want to share some of that love with you. I invite you to my kitchen table to share in two of my favourite winter recipes: my grandmother's bread and the ultimate gingerbread biscuits.

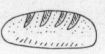 Grannie-Jo's bread

My grandmother, Grannie-Jo, made bread so often that when, aged 12, I asked her for the recipe, she looked at me a little blankly. So intuitive was her breadmaking that the concept of a recipe was long gone. In the end, I grabbed a notebook and watched her make it, asking how much a handful of something weighed and generally slowing down the process. As with everything in our relationship, Grannie-Jo displayed endless patience, and soon I had a scrap of paper with hastily scribbled scrawl covering it, which detailed her bread recipe. I rediscovered that scrap of paper many years later when I moved house, finding it tucked into the pages of a recipe book. After deciphering my pre-teen handwriting, I decided it would be the first thing I baked in my new home. I steeled myself, but cried nonetheless, as the scent of my childhood filled the air, and I took the first bite of a warm, wholesome slice. I now make this bread so often I could do it in my sleep. It made me smile when I also had to stop and think, 'Wait, what's the recipe?' when it came to writing it down. So here it is, from my kitchen to yours, with love.

Makes 1 large loaf
450g eight-grain flour
115g brown bread flour

115g strong white bread flour, plus extra for dusting

a small handful of bran

1 x 7g sachet of fast-acting yeast

a pinch of caster sugar

a pinch of salt

60ml vegetable oil

440ml warm water (measure the oil first, then top up with water until you reach the 500ml mark)

1) In a large bowl, mix together the flours, bran, yeast, sugar and salt, making sure to disperse the yeast evenly throughout.
2) Mix in the water and oil and knead for 10 minutes.
3) Cover with lightly oiled clingfilm and a tea towel and leave in a warm spot to rise for 30 minutes.
4) Knead again for 10 minutes.
5) Return the bowl to the warm spot, cover and allow to rise for another 30 minutes. Once 20 minutes have passed, preheat your oven to 220–240°C/425–475°F (temperature will very much depend on your oven, but you need to go a little hotter than your standard 'cook it in the oven' temp. I find my perfect temperature is 220°C/475°F.
6) Lightly knock out the air, shape the dough into a loaf, dust with flour all over, including both ends, and put into a 2lb/900g loaf tin. Bake for 25 minutes.

7) After 25 minutes, tip out of the tin and cook directly on the oven shelf for 5 minutes.
8) Rest on a wire rack and allow to cool before slicing (attempting to slice whilst the loaf is still hot will cause it to fall apart).
9) Enjoy simply with butter.

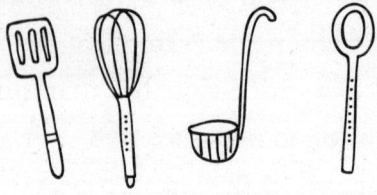

The ultimate gingerbread biscuits

This recipe has never let me down. It's a recipe that speaks of easy catch-ups, cradling mugs of tea and laughing with friends. I often make these biscuits at a point in winter when I am craving close connection and one-on-one chats, and I invite people over to share them with me. These biscuits hold their shape really well, so you can use whatever cutter you have to hand and even make edible seasonal decorations with them. They also make a cracking dunker, so I really recommend sampling with a cuppa made in your favourite mug. I hope this recipe brings you warming hugs and cosy moments.

Makes 20–30 biscuits depending on size of cutters

75g light brown soft sugar

2 tbsp golden syrup

1 tbsp black treacle

1 tsp ground cinnamon

2 tsp ground ginger

finely grated zest of 1 small orange

2.5cm piece of fresh root ginger, finely grated (optional – only add if you like the slightly fierier kick of fresh ginger)

100g butter

½ tsp bicarbonate of soda

225g plain flour

1) Preheat your oven to 180°C/160°C fan/350°F.
2) In a large saucepan, mix together the sugar, syrup, treacle, 1 tbsp water, spices, zest and fresh ginger over a medium heat. Keep stirring to avoid the sugars catching on the bottom of the pan.
3) Once combined and boiling, add the butter and remove from the heat.
4) When the butter has melted, add the bicarbonate of soda and flour and mix thoroughly to create a smooth dough.
5) Transfer to a plate, cover and place in the fridge to chill and harden (30–60 minutes).
6) Once the dough is firm, roll out on a floured surface until 3–5mm thick (depending on preference).
7) Use your cutter and begin to cut out your biscuit shapes, transferring them to baking trays lined with parchment or baking paper. Note there is no need to grease the paper. Space the cookies slightly apart, as they may spread whilst cooking.
8) Bake in the oven for 10–15 minutes until lightly golden and firm.
9) Once out of the oven, leave the biscuits to cool on the baking trays for 5 minutes, then transfer to a wire rack

to cool completely. (Note the biscuits will harden as they cool).
10) Stick the kettle on and put your feet up as you enjoy with your favourite cuppa – bliss!

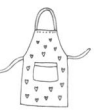 ## Activity: Create a cosy cooking retreat

Creating a cosy cooking retreat for yourself can turn the chore of cooking into a mindful and blissful experience. The sense of hygge that exists in my kitchen is aided not just by what I cook but *how* I cook. I cook with intention and patience, and I create pockets of time that are just for me.

Take a moment to consider what you would love to cook. What needs to happen in your cooking retreat? Do you want the whole family involved, or do you want some time alone with your favourite music playing? What dish would make your soul happy? What would make your tastebuds zing?

Gather everything you need. Source your ingredients and dig out any cooking pots, dishes or utensils you want to hand so you don't disrupt your calm cooking retreat to rootle around in the back of a cupboard or make a last-minute dash to the shops.

Then consider what you will do whilst your dishes cook. Perhaps you will sit at your kitchen table, notepad in front of you, and daydream, scribbling hopes, plans and ambitions that cook, bake and develop along with the food you prepare? Perhaps you will curl up with a favourite book? Or maybe you will enjoy what my mother calls 'chef's perks' and snaffle a few freshly baked biccies before they're gobbled up!

Whatever it is, taking time to create a cosy winter cooking retreat is another way to relax into the seasonal energy. Plan it now, put it in the diary, protect that time just for you and enjoy cooking in tune with winter.

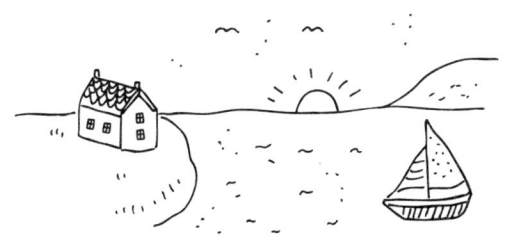

Chapter 9: Winter's light

We associate winter with darkness, but there is such beauty in winter's light. Light plays an enormous role in winter, starting with the awakening glory of sunrise through to the glowing embers of sunset. From fairy lights to candlelight to flickering flames dancing in fireplaces, winter showcases many levels of light, highlighting the energy that exists in each lumen.

If you have ever wondered why the sky is blue (or tried to confidently answer that query from a child in the back seat), the answer is Rayleigh scattering. Rayleigh scattering is the process where certain atmospheric substances like nitrogen and oxygen deflect blue and violet light. As we have a lot of oxygen and nitrogen in our atmosphere, we have a lot of blue and violet light deflected back at us, thus creating a bright blue sky.

Contrary to simple childhood drawings of a large yellow circle, sunlight is made up of all seven colours of the rainbow (red, orange, yellow, green, blue, indigo and violet) and all of them have different wavelengths. Blue and green colours have shorter wavelengths and red and orange have longer wavelengths. At sunrise and sunset, sunlight with all its colours has to travel through more atmosphere to reach our eyes and this means the shorter wavelengths are filtered out, leaving only the vibrant reds and oranges we associate with sunrise and sunset.

Winter sunrises and sunsets are the most glorious of the year, noted for their exceptionally deep and vibrant colours. There are several reasons why winter offers us the most spectacular aerial display, including the fact that there is less atmospheric pollution. Dust, pollen and air pollution can all lessen the intensity of colour. As any hay fever sufferer will gratefully tell you, these allergens are much reduced in winter, meaning the air is cleaner for winter light to shine through with more intensity. The notion of 'hazy summer days' goes for the weather too. There is a literal haze preventing us from viewing the full spectrum of colours until winter allows us to see the sun rise and set in all its unfiltered splendour.

Winter is also a less humid season. The concept of winter humidity was introduced to me by my friend Bruce, a Canadian who endures far wilder winters than I have ever known. I'd never come across the idea of winter humidity before but it works in the same way as summer humidity; it is how much water vapour is in the air around us. It explains why we feel colder in the 10°C temperature of December than the 0°C of January. The moisture in the air around us means we feel the cold damp seep into our bones, leaving behind a chill that feels impossible to shake off. January through March offers more crisp, clear, glistening mornings. Mornings where you can see your breath and feel your cheeks pinken. Whilst we may feel the cold air around us, it is easier to stay warm and cosy within our coats, whereas a damp, humid day sees us hurpling (hunched with cold). Humidity or moisture in the air also dulls colours, and so the reward on a dry, crisp winter morning is a vibrant winter sunrise. Winter sunsets also have a unique seasonal vividity due to the angle of the sun. During winter, the sun sits lower in the sky. The lower the sun, the more atmosphere the wavelengths have to work through, which again filters out the blues and greens and leaves only the coppers and fires on display. As the angle of the earth's tilt lengthens, so does the amount of time the sun takes to set, allowing us to notice the sunset and enjoy it for much longer.[1]

Although the term 'sunrise' conjures up visions of 5am starts, life is a lot more civilized in winter. Unlike my partner, a professional photographer who will get out of bed at 3am if necessary to capture the perfect light, I am, wombling aside, less likely to leave the snuggly comfort of my duvet in the early hours. Winter offers us the gift of a far more accessible sunrise. In mid-January, the sun wakes to greet us at around 8am. This later start makes being present for sunrise a lot more achievable, and it is so very worth it. These sunrises are unveiled daily just for us, if we take the time to look up. I like to imagine the winter sun sleeping through its alarm clock, then rushing into the day, hastily shaking off the velvet shawl of darkness and offering truly spectacular colours to make up for its tardiness.

The sunrises and sunsets are definitely one of the characteristics of winter that I appreciate the most. To start and end our day with such beauty serves as a reminder of something bigger and more powerful than us. Heading into our day, we can look up and see sunrises beckoning us into the possibilities of the day ahead, whilst sunsets remind us that no matter what has happened in our day, there is always something beautiful to be found.

If you haven't paid attention to the sunrise or sunset for a while, consider spending some time with the winter sun. There is a wide window of opportunity for sunrise in winter, as between January and March the sun will gradually get up over two hours earlier, with a mid-March sunrise occurring around 6am. Even if you just do it once every winter, it is worth getting up to connect and recharge yourself with the winter light. If you can take some quiet time in the evening to wind down your day, again between early January and the end of March the time of sunset will get 3.5 hours later, so there is an opportunity to weave it into your diary no matter your schedule.

A really beautiful activity (weather permitting) is to plan to see the last sunset in winter, either according to the spring equinox or according to your own rewrite of your year. This is a time to bid farewell to winter, something which we'll look at in more detail in our final chapter, and a last opportunity to simply acknowledge this beautiful season after three whole months of restoration and recharging. It is a wonderful moment to reflect on all that winter has brought you and what you are carrying from one season into the next.

Of course, sunlight is just one aspect and we can draw inspiration from multiple traditions to celebrate all light in winter.

A festival of winter light

The word 'festival' can feel synonymous with summer. The sunshine, the dancing, throwing our arms in the air, feeling our skin tighten after too long being baked in the rays, and a sense of freedom, escape and fun. It can be hard to imagine a festival in winter because the energy and the environment are so removed from that sunny summer feel. However, winter can be the perfect backdrop for a different kind of festival. A festival with a more nourishing and soulful vibe that really supports our feelings of expansion and freedom, in a season that has traditionally been sold to us as claustrophobic or stifling but needn't be seen as either.

Candles feature heavily in my winter. I light them during my winter retreats, on my hygge days and continually swap harsh overhead lights for the gentle glow of a burning flame. I use candles throughout winter to connect me to the season and they serve as a visual reminder of the part of the year I'm in. Candles also serve a deeper and more spiritual purpose, being used in festivals as a way to mark an intention or an energy shift, or to highlight a particular ritual or element of celebration. The use of candlelight is shared across multiple festivals that are hosted in winter.

For example, in Kwanzaa, a week of celebrating African

culture with friends, families and communities, a candle is lit every day on the *kinara* (candle holder) for that day's principle. The candle provides a symbolism and literal illumination of the focus of that day's celebration. This festival, taking place as it does right at the start of winter, is a gorgeous reminder of the importance of people and connection. It seems fitting that it takes place at the very start of the season that encourages the same.

Diwali, also known as the festival of lights, uses candles as a symbol of light over darkness, good over evil, knowledge over ignorance. The festival gets its name from the row (*avali*) of clay lamps (*deepa*) that are lit outside homes to symbolize the inner light that protects from spiritual darkness.

Hanukkah, celebrated by millions of Jews worldwide, is an eight-day festival, with each day of celebration beginning with the lighting of candles in a menorah, to commemorate the miracle of light.

Beginning before Christmas, Christians light four candles across each Sunday of Advent, which represent hope, peace, joy and love.

The Chinese Lantern Festival takes place on the 15th day of the first lunar month, two weeks after Lunar New Year, and marks both the first full moon of the new lunar year and the end of the new year period. The lighting of lanterns highlights a time for reconciliation, peace and forgiveness, letting go of the previous year and moving into the new one.

All of these winter festivals invite us to appreciate, reflect and enjoy all light, from the full moon to the tiniest tea light. The meaning behind even one single flame is powerful and impactful. There is a reminder in these tiny lights that even small actions are significant.

We don't need huge bursts or reserves of energy to burn bright; a whole room can be lit by a single tea light. The same is true of our actions in winter. Even the smallest energetic shift can change an entire day or mood. If we arrive into winter feeling exhausted or as though we need to rest, that's OK. We can gently and easily move through winter, achieving what we need to, with tiny lights sparkling, twinkling and guiding our way through the season. Every action we take, no matter how small, is the metaphorical lighting of another tealight, switching on another fairy bulb, illuminating our own path. If we don't have the energy to dazzle with floodlights, it doesn't mean we have to sit in the dark. This is not a still or stagnant season; these smaller acts and softer lights represent the gentle energy that pulses through winter.

Small energy moments

There is something truly satisfying about completing small acts by utilizing that gentle thrum of winter energy. One of my favourites of these small bursts of activity in winter is cleaning my car. In itself it's not a remarkable feat but, having lived in a first-floor apartment for 10 years with no access to an outdoor tap, the ability to now clean my own car still makes me happy.

From observation, I would estimate that 90% of cars in winter wear a grimy overcoat, woven by the salt, dirt and mud on the roads. I can't deny the small glow of accomplishment I feel every time I spot my newly gleaming car. It is a tiny act, it is a small tealight, it is not even a priority in the maelstrom of other tasks demanding my attention. But this one tiny act is an example of tapping into the gentle energy of winter. Achieving something that doesn't require a huge energetic push but that still changes the tone for the rest of the season.

Small wins and pleasures often get ignored or pushed back to the spring and summer seasons, when we can combine them with multiple other activities and have a whole day of productivity. Yet how much more meaningful are small energetic acts in winter. These gentle actions are a great antidote to the constant pressure of doing and the ingrained resistance we can feel to stopping. As I touched on earlier, we may wistfully envy those creatures who hibernate throughout winter, but we are not designed for it. It is very hard to simply stop and do nothing. We are all embroiled in a culture that prioritizes doing and hustling, and the thought of coming to a standstill can be jarring. However, we don't need to grind to a halt in winter, nor do we need to move at an aggressive pace. Winter is the season of gentle progress, to tune in and reflect on what we want to achieve and why. It is a time to plan the how, without needing the energy to tackle and accomplish everything all at once.

The gentle winter light illuminates what really matters to

us. We can often feel a resistance to winter because we want to do so much but cannot find the energy and so feel trapped in our frustration and inability to complete. What if we didn't need to race towards the finish line but instead could stroll at a steady pace, allowing us to enjoy the journey and spend time with each task? Instead of expending huge amounts of energy blitzing the entire house, we could tidy one drawer, one shelf, one nook at a time. Instead of attempting to write a whole novel, we could write one sentence per day and take time to reflect on the story we want to tell. It is these gentle acts of energy, these micro-illuminations, that help us build and restore our energy reserves in winter. Not rushing but always moving forwards.

Winter is not about total darkness or total cessation of activity. Winter isn't a time for total anything. But it is the perfect time for an energetic shift, and leaning into gentle winter light is a great way to move through the season. We can build and navigate our own path through winter using the light and energy that it provides. If we wait until the floodlights go back on, i.e. sit still and wait for summer, then we are in for a frustrating and disappointing year and we won't get to enjoy our much-anticipated summer, as it will be full of all the tasks and activities that we put on ice during the coldest season. Instead of stopping, pave your pathway with winter energy and embrace winter light to guide you.

The start of lighter days and brighter skies

Winter brings the gift of light. As soon as winter arrives on the solstice, the days start becoming longer, moving us towards lighter and brighter days. Far from the associations with darkness, winter offers a gentle glow of light, which increasingly brightens throughout the season until it spotlights the start of spring. This gradual glow provides an internal awakening. It's as though there is a bulb in our core and winter increases the brightness just a little more with each day. We feel the warmth, light and energy grow inside us, illuminating areas that have felt dark or depressing, brightening our thoughts and spirits, banishing shadows and showing us there is nothing to fear in the year ahead.

The knowledge that winter is the start of lighter days can offer a really useful framework for our thoughts and reflections. Each extra moment of brightness, each extra minute of light, reminds us to look for the glimmers, to seek out the gifts and make the most of this beautiful season.

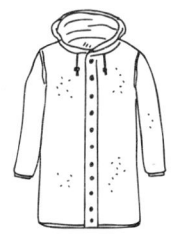

Chapter 10:
Getting out in winter

I'm a country girl at heart, but if there is one time of year when I really appreciate a city, it's in winter.

I used to live in Oxford, which I consider a gateway city: it offers an introduction to the convenience and variety of city life, without the pressure and intensity of, say, London. With its history, gardens and parks, alongside restaurants, shops and spires, it really is a blend of beauty and bustle.

Although I loved living in Oxford, it could be overwhelming at times. Oxford attracts over 7 million visitors every year and the architecture and facilities don't always seem to cope well with this swell of bodies, especially in the summer. People are everywhere. Every single café is stuffed to the brim, the simple act of buying a coffee can turn into a (literal) bun fight. Like many UK cities, the infrastructure simply doesn't work well in the heat. There is little effective ventilation, courtyards are full of crowds and walking tours and every purchase seems a little swollen with tourist tax. It is impossible to walk in a straight line as you weave, duck and dodge your way around tourists pointing cameras in every direction.

Although cities positively teem with people in the summer, it is the season when I find them the most lonely. No one really has time for you in the summer; you are just another person, making another demand on an over-stretched hospitality industry. It feels as though cities don't have space. There's nowhere to sit, nowhere to go, nowhere to *be*. Places you want to eat in are fully booked, tables are all occupied or being aggressively man-marked. However, once winter arrives, it is as though cities catch their breath and deeply exhale.

Without a jostling queue, people have time to exchange a few words. You can start a conversation with strangers, knowing that they aren't trying to sell you a hop-on/hop-off bus tour. People seem to decompress and laugh more with each other. There are pockets of welcome warmth everywhere, both the physical kind from shops and cafés, but also the emotional kind, as people take the time to reconnect with each other.

Don't get me wrong, I love that Oxford and cities around the UK attract visitors. Part of what makes Oxford so beautiful is the range of quirky independent retailers which simply couldn't exist without the economic boost of tourism. But I only ever really connect with cities in winter. I felt I could really see Oxford then, uncover hidden gems that were tucked away down smaller alleys, inviting exploration. I used to walk to work in the mornings and witness the city waking up. It was my favourite time of day. The bright, crisp morning sunshine spotlighting different points of architecture and history, drawing the eye to something special.

I do understand why it's tempting to stay huddled indoors. When the weather is grey and uninviting and we have everything at our fingertips courtesy of food and parcel delivery services, we can ask ourselves 'why bother?' when it comes to going out in winter. But we have to be *in* winter to really experience the magic.

Walking (the dogs) in a winter wonderland

Along with the many other heart-sparks of joy that come with having dogs, my eyes were truly opened to the beauty of winter thanks to Bella and Darcy, my two black cockapoos (joyfully known as 'spoodles' in Australia), who require walking three times per day. We do longer early morning strides and post-dinner ambles, with a lunchtime walk around the block thrown in to stretch our legs and provide a very welcome screen-break (for me, not them).

Of course, some days this feels far from ideal. In the pitch-black darkness, with tendrils of hair soaked by biblical rain being whipped against my face by a howling wind, I do question my life choices. Could I overcome my allergies and become a cat person after all? But here's the thing. Those windy, rainy and frankly dismal dog walks don't really happen in winter. Remember autumn with the beautiful changing leaves which we all love so much? That's the keeper of the muddiest, wettest and chilliest dog walks. It is the autumnal months that see us arrive home to embark on a frenzied towelling, desperately trying to pre-empt the inevitable nose-to-tail shake that will redecorate the hallway in fetching splodges of sludge.

Winter walks are entirely different. Beauty and cold combine to literally take your breath away. Morning dog walks in winter see me and the girls pad our way through a world covered in what the environmentalist writer Roger Deakin described as a sharp, sugaring frost.[1] Our surroundings look as though a shimmery kiss has been bestowed by a Hollywood starlet. That kiss of glitter remains until the sun warms and melts the covering of scattered diamonds that don the grass, frost the windowsills and encrust every leaf.

Winter walks drum the beauty of nature's heartbeat into our souls with every step, but we have to be outside to connect with it. All the magic and wonder of winter walking was hidden from me until we acquired our first dog, Bella. I say 'acquired' because she originally belonged to my father-in-law, Terry. When he had to go into hospital with a leg injury, we agreed to have Bella to stay for a few days . . . that was over five years ago. Although he healed well, Terry no longer had the mobility to regularly walk a dog and so she settled into our household (and she has regular cuddle visits with Tez, so everyone is happy).

Walking Bells was a huge contributor to me falling in love with winter. I had to walk her regardless of temperature or rainfall or daylight. When you've gotta go, you've gotta go and when a dog needs to go, that means a human is following behind them. Bella was my introduction to a very different side of winter.

Seeing my dog's black nose smattered with frost, making her look as though she'd nose-dived into icing sugar, made me giggle. Seeing her sheer confusion and delight the first time she put her paws in snow, and then tried to shake it off as the dobbles[2] stubbornly clung to her fur, creating some fairly stylish snow boots, melted my heart. Even as we both slipped and slid our way home along paths which were yet to be graced by a gritter, I was smiling. I was observing. I was *seeing* winter. Bella's fascination was contagious and I adopted her mindful curiosity. We crumped over the ice-encrusted leaves and listened to the animals safely tucked away in their subnivium beneath the snow. All of this delighted Bella and enchanted me and I realized that this was the first time I had regularly been outside in winter in decades.

Why had I never noticed this before?

Typically, in previous jobs, I would have already been at work for quite some time before the sun rolled out of bed, stretched across the horizon and began its day's work. Similarly, I would often finish after sunset, meaning entire working weeks could pass without me seeing any more of the sun than a glimpse through the window, if I remembered to look up. I didn't think it bothered me. After all, I didn't like winter and I didn't want to spend any time in it, so I didn't believe I was missing anything. But my seasonal affective disorder made the darkness tough. Days seemed indistinguishable and weeks blurred into each other, resulting in a feeling of never-ending trudge. The winter of 2020 changed all that.

At first I didn't actually notice the impact of not commuting. I was too preoccupied with the pandemic and its very severe impact on the company I was working for at the time. What I did gradually notice, however, was that for the first winter in years I didn't feel *that* bad. When checking in with my mood, dipping a very cautious toe into the depths of my winter mind, I found to my surprised relief that I was OK. The mires of depression I had come to expect and dread weren't there. I felt OK. Actually, I felt good. What on earth was going on? This was a time when feeling utterly miserable would have been not only understandable but completely supported by others. The world was on fire and yet here I was feeling OK.

Now, I should clarify, I don't mean I was feeling OK about the pandemic. There was plenty of worry and anxiety in the world and I was far from immune from it. But the crippling and debilitating depression that had become my companion throughout winter simply wasn't there. On realizing this, I felt joyous and deeply suspicious in equal measure. Anyone who has ever struggled with their mental health will tell you that you never really relax into the good times. It is hard to enjoy them because you are always waiting for the other shoe to drop. Waiting for something to change. Waiting to wake up the next day with a completely different mood and a new challenge to face. Yet, that winter, it wasn't there. So, what had changed? What had happened to me? Why was I feeling so different?

What was different was that I was *in* winter. Not watching it through my hastily demisted windscreen, office window or train carriage. I wasn't in it for 30 seconds between tube dashes. I wasn't in it just long enough to curse the cold before bowling back onto the underground and heading for an overheated office. I was properly *in* winter and living in alignment *with* winter.

Without an outrageous commute to complete, I was regularly walking Bella in full morning daylight. This introduced me to winter in a way I couldn't imagine. I walked further, noticed more, laughed with people as we clutched coffees and stamped our feet in a bid to keep warm. I let children delay their entrance through the school gates just a few precious moments longer via a quick wave hello to Bella, who was more than happy to tail-wag back. I was (safely) engaging with my community, and given the times we were in, a kind word, a smile, a 'good morning' was more impactful than ever. Moreover, rather than dragging a still-sleepy Bella around the block, trying to hastily squeeze in a comfort walk before leaving for work, we strolled companionably. I had time. I had daylight. I felt happiness.

I *hate* when wellness advice favours the privileged and I fully appreciate this particular alignment with winter won't be an option for everyone. In the majority of my jobs, I have had zero control over my diary and no option to work morning daylight into my routine. However, this experience did confirm what we know in our souls. Working with, not against, winter is the answer. It made me happy. It made me well. It made me question how I had been approaching winter up until this point. Even small tweaks and adjustments can align us better with winter and it is worth thinking about what we can change for a short few months of the year and put into practice, whether during or outside of the working week.

Once I realized the difference it was making to my mood when living in alignment with winter, I knew I couldn't return to battling it. I didn't want to. In spending time in winter, really noticing the season in all its glory, I was spellbound by the beauty. The only sadness I felt that year was that I hadn't noticed it sooner. I had been so busy blocking winter out on my scuttle from house, to car, to office and back again, that I never noticed the sheer astonishing loveliness that was all around me. Not only had I not noticed it, I'd been actively avoiding it, but as soon as I accepted it, I felt better. Happier. Comforted. That year, I was really *in* winter and I loved it. More so, in aligning with winter, I had more energy and found the season recharged rather than depleted me. There was an energy in winter air that I had never noticed before and I was keen to utilize it.

If ever I consider winter a lethargic or sluggish season, my dogs provide a very real reminder that the exact opposite is true. My dogs get bolder in winter. They become more intrepid on their walks. They have extra zest and a little extra sass, as though they recognize that this is the time for their black fur coats to shine. They appear buoyed up by winter, excited by new smells and pull to investigate a bush or a flower, which in turn brings those treasures to my attention and I can share in the wonder of winter with them.

The winter zest

I have an aunt for whom the solution to most problems is a brisk walk along Dún Laoghaire pier. If you've never been, Dún Laoghaire (pronounced 'Done-Leer-ee') is a suburban coastal town in southern Ireland and it has two piers, both just shy of a mile long, which are to my aunt's mind the answer to everything. Heartbroken? Hungry? Bored? Tired? A brisk walk down Dún Laoghaire pier and you'll be sorted. Whilst we might be quick to dismiss the benefits of bracing (read freezing) fresh air as an old wives' tale, actually it turns out there is something in it.

Although not always tempting, getting our bodies cold has multiple benefits. The recent rise in popularity of open-water swimming is largely due to the recognition that there are mental health benefits of reducing our body's temperature. Cold-water immersion has been linked to an enhanced positive mood state[3] with individuals showing higher perceived psycho-physical wellbeing[4] and significant improvements in mood disorders.[5]

Whole-body exposure to cold triggers a release of neurotransmitters such as serotonin, cortisol, dopamine, norepinephrine and endorphins, all of which play a significant role in stress management, mood and emotional regulation.[6]

However, although the impacts on the brain are significant, you don't need to put your face or head under the water in order to get the benefits. The research has been conducted on what is known as 'whole-body head-out' exposure. Sitting or standing in cold water, or swimming with your head above the water will see you find your zest and can be a lot more comfortable than fully dunking under.

There are several theories on how long you need to be exposed to the cold in order to get the benefits, with some arguing that the longer you are in the cold, the more benefit you will experience. However, the neuroscience doesn't support this, as there is a natural plateau in the impacts and benefits, so you don't need to be in the cold for ages. The exact time will depend on temperature, body size and composition; there is no one-size-fits-all. What is recommended is a slow build, starting with 30-second to 1-minute exposures and building up. It's always important to consider your own medical history and seek expert opinion before taking the plunge.

If you're unsure if regularly getting cold is for you, then research shows there can be benefits from a single one-time exposure. You can also get a similar hormone release from taking a cold shower, so if the thought of a dip in a lake literally turns you cold, then perhaps play with cold water therapy by gradually adjusting your shower to cool, with a blast of cold for the final minute. Getting cold holds more appeal when you can immediately wrap yourself up in a soft and fluffy towel and get warm and dry, but there is no doubt that the sense of community and camaraderie plays a huge part in why open-water swimming is so popular. The shared experience of doing something that may appear to others to be just a little bit bonkers is indescribable. Also, the buzz and hubbub when you emerge is palpable, the air around you filled with laughter.

You don't even need to be fully exposed to the cold to feel the benefits. The lakeside chatter reminds me of spilling into steamy cafés on a trip to Iceland, everyone talking nineteen to the dozen and laughing loudly as they stripped off outdoor layers and acclimatized to the warm environment around them. Although fully dressed, with no danger of even an inch of skin being exposed to the below-freezing chill, there were still huge benefits of being in the cold and dropping our core body temperature. It brought a sense of exhilaration, a feeling of truly being alive, and it was joyful. We can absorb some of the winter zest and be invigorated by the energy. Feeling lethargic and sluggish? Follow my aunt's advice and get cold; you'll feel amazing for it.

Of course, winter doesn't just offer us the cold. We also get the gift of apricity, a perfect word which describes the warmth of the sun on a winter's day. The physiological effects of sunshine are well proven; our mood diminishes without it and we experience a welcome flood of the feel-good hormone serotonin when basking in the rays. Apricity is extra special, as to experience it, you are outside *in* winter. To feel the sun unexpectedly warm your bones on a winter's day is a new level of happiness.

When we connect with nature and the zest of winter, we can fully recharge ourselves; mind, body and soul. The beautiful word 'chibbly' describes something being crisp or crackly with frost. I believe the energy of winter can be chibbly. Crisp, crackling, electric. The very air is alive with an energy that we miss out on when we hide away and cocoon ourselves inside. Winter is a season that encourages you to be present, to notice every detail of your day, right down to your breath, which is reflected back to you in puffs of condensation. Winter shows us that which is so easy to ignore when we are busy and marching through our day. That sense of presence truly is a gift of winter.

What to do on miserable weather days

Of course, not every day in winter will bring apricity, blue skies and crisp frosts. It is still important to be *in* winter, even when the weather isn't inviting us outdoors. We need a plan to cope with the more miserable of weather.

1. **Accept where you are.** If it is lashing down with rain, then know you are going to get wet and don your wellies. However, the first two months of winter (January and February) are typically the driest, so you should have some great opportunities to get outside, ahead of any early spring rainfall.
2. **Set yourself up with a plan,** an idea or an agenda for the walk. Are you going to wrap up warm and

visit your favourite coffee house? Your favourite bookshop? Could you meet a friend? If you are walking somewhere with a purpose, can you give yourself a reward such as listening to your favourite album or catching up on episodes of a much-loved podcast en route? Or can you give yourself headspace by experiencing only the walk and nothing else?

3. **Find your spaces.** I will always be drawn to words and so one of my go-to places in winter is the library. In a world driven by consumerism, there is something beautiful about libraries being the last place where you can spend hours of your time and not be expected to spend any money. Moreover, there are a multitude of activities for adults and children which are free to attend. Everything from book clubs and discussion groups to crafting and language schools. These are spaces to meet people and have meaningful conversations, to create or learn and to be together. Spaces to be warm and feel part of a community, and it's all for free. If you hold a hangover of a belief about deathly quiet and intimidating spaces, then know that libraries are a different breed these days. Gone is the aggressive shushing and demand for silence; I have witnessed indoor football tournaments and baking competitions within larger city libraries.

4. **Take advantage of off-season perks.** City spaces up and down the country do not close for the winter, but

they are easier to access, and tickets are often cheaper off-season. Many museums and galleries are free to visit and those that aren't often reduce ticket prices to attract people off-peak. There is something special about being able to move at your own pace, see the artwork, dawdle and dream as you walk around. Or indeed lead your kids through these spaces without fear of losing sight of them in a large crowd. There is more liberty and more freedom in cities in the winter and it is a beautiful feeling to explore them accordingly. Given there are many more options and buildings in cities, there is opportunity for fun and adventure, whatever your age. Cosiness can be found everywhere. Fireplaces roaring in cafés and pubs. Rooftop bars with heaters and blankets to keep you snug as you observe the world from a height. Take advantage of the wriggle room of the season and the off-peak perks it provides.

5. **Commit and go.** I find the most beneficial walks are the ones where, just beforehand, I am sat inside looking out at the grey clouds and thinking how uninspiring the world looks. When it is tempting to stay indoors because the world looks drab, I will grab my boots and deliberately go and look for inspiration or beauty. It is rarely truly grey and miserable. Once outside, we can see the glittering frosts and cobwebs laced with ice crystals. It is a season of diamonds

scattered underneath your feet that dance and sparkle in the light. On darker and gloomier days, it is inevitably brighter and more inviting outside than it looks through a window pane. On many occasions, you'll experience a 'foxing day', where the weather is much better than anticipated and the day turns out far better than predicted. These are the days when the rewards of getting outside are greatest.

6. **Remember it is worth it.** Of course, this approach isn't just for winter, this is an all-season toolkit, especially if your part of the world is experiencing continually unpredictable weather. But winter is the season that reminds us it is worth our efforts. It is worth stepping outside. To really discover winter, we need to be in it. We need to go out, explore and experience all the elements of winter and observe what nature is offering. Accepting and enjoying, being present and really truly engaging with winter meant I fell in love with winter walking, wherever I was. I hope you can too.

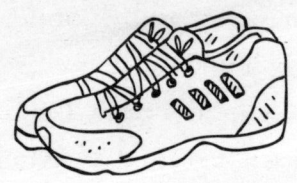

Chapter 11:
Moving through winter

In winter, 61% of Brits stop exercising altogether.[1] Many of us blame the cold for this downshift in motivation and movement. I know myself that sometimes the thought of getting changed, or getting sweaty, when there is a chill in the air can be less than appealing. That said, there is more to our reluctance to move than just the temperature. We can be so hard on ourselves and cross with our own lack of motivation, but it's important to know that dropping exercise when the conditions get a little harder is *not* inherent laziness on our part, but rather symptomatic of the world we live in.

The amygdala is the alarm bell of the brain, the over-reactive part. I often describe the amygdala as the office temp: lovely, very enthusiastic but doesn't really understand the business. When we are in a state of stress, our responses can be overrun by the amygdala. This state of amygdala takeover is known as 'amygdala hijack' and we cannot make good decisions in this state. Your amygdala doesn't really care about future you; it only focuses on what feels good now. Whereas going for a run may benefit future you, the amygdala will counter that sitting on the sofa with some chocolate and binge-watching a boxset will feel better now. It can therefore derail and demotivate you into staying put and not moving. If the weather looks unappealing or the temperature feels a little chilly, then the amygdala will happily convince you to stay still and stay toasty, ignoring any potential health and mood gains to be had from exercise.

It is not our fault that we are in amygdala hijack. Modern living is increasingly stressful for the brain, as we are overloaded with information at a rate that we were never designed to process. Everything from 24-hour news through to doomscrolling, means our brains are trying to process information at a far greater rate than is manageable, leaving us feeling overwhelmed and indecisive.

If you've ever been getting ready to go out, only to find yourself sitting on the end of your bed staring into space, then you know that sense of overwhelm we live with, day in, day out. Our brains literally don't know what to do next and we have to pause whilst they catch up. Enter the amygdala, making poor decisions for future you that feel great now. Although the amygdala may not care about the longer-term benefits of exercise, the rest of us should. Exercise can mitigate the impact of stress and calm our amygdala down, lifting us out of amygdala hijack and into a better physical and emotional state.

Our other most commonly cited reason for not exercising is lack of time, but there is nearly always time to be found.

We spend 22% more time on our devices in winter than at any other time of the year. In fact, research conducted by retailer Sports Direct showed that over the weeks of winter, we will spend 441 hours, that's 3 hours per day, scrolling through social media videos and online memes alone.[2] It is worth pointing out that this research was completed *before* the ubiquitous rise of apps such as TikTok and the manipulation of algorithms to keep a tight grip on our attention. Whilst 33% of us reassure ourselves with the excuse 'I'll go tomorrow',[3] the way we live and the increased scrolling combined with the additional stresses of the festivities can make movement unlikely in winter. A downturn in activity leads to a downturn in mood.

We mustn't be hard on ourselves if we are struggling to move through winter; it makes sense. Instead of worrying about our outputs, we should try reviewing our inputs. We need to consider what information we are trying to process and look at how exercise can support us. A simple 20-minute walk around the block can reduce cortisol (stress hormone) levels, leading to a better mood and a more positive outlook. You've probably heard of fight or flight stress responses and it's worth noting that both of these responses involve movement. Our bodies are designed to move when stressed. If you're able to, try getting more movement into your day, especially if you feel overwhelmed. The movement can be anything that gets your heart rate up and leaves you feeling as though you've exerted a little effort. Swap 20 minutes of scrolling for 20 minutes of movement and monitor the difference in your mood.

The multiple benefits of movement

Exercise has such a plethora of benefits. It's often sold to us as purely aesthetic, an appearance equation. Do this + eat this = you'll look like this. But the benefits of exercise go deeper than surface level, and the impact on our mood is by far the greatest advantage. There isn't a lot in modern living that stimulates our brain the way it was designed to be used. We are creatures who need to physically move, and we feel the impacts of sitting still for too long. We get stiff, sore and tense when we don't move around, yet so many of us lead very sedentary lives, particularly in winter. Research into the average Brit's winter habits, which one can assume are not so very different to other northern hemisphere inhabitants, shows that we will spend 42% more time sedentary over winter. That's an additional six hours per day across the season where we will sit still instead of moving around.[4] That's going to take its toll.

We need to move through winter for our mental health and for our mood management. If we are prone to the winter blues or the more impactful SAD, then movement changes from a nice-to-have to a seasonal essential. A number of recent studies show that physical exercise provides an effective and easily accessible treatment for patients suffering from SAD.[5] In fact, exercise may be one of the largest components of facilitating effective treatment for SAD. Incorporating exercise as part of your regular SAD treatment, along with light therapy and vitamin D supplementation, can be a seasonal adjustment that sets you up for your year ahead.

Exercise is a confidence booster and we can use that boost throughout winter as we reassess our ambitions, goals and desires. In a HIIT (high intensity interval training) class I attended, the trainer told the class, 'If you stop doing things when they become hard, then that becomes your norm. You need to do hard things to remind yourself that you can.' This is so true. We need to continually challenge our brain to boost our confidence and remind ourselves of what we are capable of. When we do challenging things, we are able to overcome more challenges. In winter when we do less, move less, challenge ourselves less, if we aren't careful, this can lead to us feeling uncertain and lacking in confidence. We won't rise into our day so much as hesitantly take a faltering step. This can add to a feeling of low mood and helplessness in winter. Exercise can help ground us in our bodies more confidently. It can make us feel more *us* and as though we can conquer more. Exercising in winter is a powerful tool to manage our winter mood, but it does require a little planning.

One challenge to moving through winter is the darkness. Not only does this have practical implications, but can also impact our ongoing motivation and enthusiasm. If you drive to and from work in the dark and don't get to see much daylight in the autumn and winter months, then each day can blur into the next, lacking distinction or definition.

Novelty helps us to feel each day is unique and memorable. Oliver Burkeman in his book *Four Thousand Weeks* describes the role of novelty playing a part in making childhood summer holidays feel blissfully endless, as every day brought something new to explore, discover or play with, and so the time felt filled.[6] However, as adults, our days tend to blur into one but it is a different sensation to time whizzing by. When days have no distinction, there is no separation, no glimmer, no sparkle. We can feel a sense of trudging through the dark from autumn onwards in a way that isn't helpful or hopeful. Literally moving our bodies, doing more, creating distinction and novelty, can help us to move through the season and to feel the season is moving forwards.

Dealing with the dark side

There is, sadly, another side of darkness, which is that it can bring limitation and intimidation. Routes that I happily walk in daylight become inaccessible to me in the dark because of fear. Parks, woods and country lanes, places that teem with people in summer but fall deathly quiet in winter, *can* offer blissful isolation and headspace but are also likely be laced with an uncomfortable feeling of risk. Any pleasure in a walk can be completely overridden by worries of being targeted or attacked and I am not alone in feeling this fear: 71% of women and over half of men surveyed said the darker nights make it difficult to find well-lit running routes, meaning they avoid exercising outside.[7] It's also hard to confidently run when worried about tree roots and potholes creating unwanted trip hazards in the dark. This can disrupt usual exercise patterns and mean that, like Jacob, my friend's husband I mentioned earlier, we stop completely and our moods darken along with the skies as we lose the mental health benefits of our regular exercise regime.

That said, when there are opportunities to be safely in the dark, there is an envelopment to winter darkness like no other. There is a velvety quality to the black, the softness contrasting with the crisp cold, like a cashmere throw laid on freshly laundered bed sheets. My favourite walks in winter are just before sunrise. I love walking into the daylight with no idea of what the day will unveil itself to be. As you know, more often than not I am accompanied by my two dogs, albeit cockapoos whose biggest threatening quality is covering the bottom of your coat with paw marks as they reach up for a cuddle. Nonetheless, I find comfort in having two creatures who by nature are related to wolves and who, I like to think, would intervene in some way should I get into trouble. That said, I am never complacent in the dark and I alter my exercise routine to accommodate the light and weather and recommend you do too. Rather than sitting out the season, we can build a new winter workout routine that forms part of our winter adjustments.

One of the best adjustments is to work out with others. Whether this is texting a friend to go for a wintery walk or joining a fitness class, there is power in the pack. It is well established that having a fitness buddy or a support network around exercise makes a huge difference. It is harder to quit when you have others holding you accountable, and the gentle peer pressure of knowing that you and your buddy are relying on each other is a big motivator.

You can also support and encourage each other when the temperature drops and there is a real sense of camaraderie in doing something together. There is another reason why a winter workout buddy is so important. This is a time of year when our brains seek connection. We want to be with others and fitness is no different. If you are able to connect with others, even if they are strangers, then your brain will thank you for that connection. Being indoors and being more sedentary means that we have less social interaction at a time of year when we want to be telling stories and connecting through meaningful conversation. Group exercise is a way to benefit body and brain in every sense.

Relaxing our routines

If you have a very rigid exercise routine then winter provides a great opportunity to shake things up and incorporate new movement. If you run or walk a few times per week but find the darker skies and the dropping temperatures are pushing you indoors, then this is the perfect time to challenge your body in a new way. Research consistently shows us that the best way to stick to exercise is to find something we love and enjoy. Winter gifts us the opportunity to try new activities, new classes, new sports. Perhaps winter is the season when you join a group dance class and shake your booty as you shake up your routine. Remember, you don't need to adjust for ever. This change in routine could be a fun way to adapt to the season and try something different. Maybe you are typically a runner but in winter you discover your inner disco diva. There are so many ways to express ourselves and move our bodies and consistently challenge ourselves, bringing benefit to mind, body and confidence.

Swapping cardio for strength training in winter is particularly beneficial, and incorporating some weightlifting into your exercise routine holds a multitude of benefits. Strength training helps you to maintain muscle mass, improve bone density and can make us more comfortable throughout the chillier days, as muscle activity generates more body heat. I notice myself that if I exercise in the morning and incorporate some strength training, then I am not affected by the temperature nearly so much. I stay warmer and more comfortable all day, not impacted by sudden drops or fluctuations in chill. Better for me, better for my heating bill.

We can be a bit scared of strength training because we imagine the weights area at the gym to be filled with super-intimidating gym bros and worry that we'll end up looking like a protein powder advert. However, strength training doesn't mean lifting weights the size of small cars, and the weights room is full of all genders and all sizes. Simple exercises incorporating small weights and body weight movements will offer the same benefits. Winter is also a good time to join because you will be in the flow of others starting New Year's resolutions. This means there will be plenty of new bodies in the gym who are not experts and you can learn together without feeling self-conscious.

Strength training is also great for your brain. It improves mental agility and executive functioning, helping us with planning, organizing and decision-making. At a time of year where making decisions and problem-solving is more difficult, our brains welcome the assistance weight-lifting can offer. Strength training also improves blood-sugar regulation, which can be really useful to help us curb cravings when we are surrounded by the sugary temptations that seem to feature around the festivities.

If you want to stop your running shoes gathering a layer of dust, then swap the pavements for the treadmill. We can consider treadmill running boring, as we are, literally, going nowhere. However, we can adjust treadmills in a multitude of ways in order to keep our run interesting. Many treadmills have pre-programmed runs with settings designed to match a video of an outdoor run. This means the incline will consistently switch it up and we can get the feel of running outdoors. Without having to worry about personal safety from traffic or others around us, we can relax into our run (as much as we ever can relax whilst running!) and turn up our playlists, watch the match or really get into an audiobook. Far from being constricting, treadmills can offer us a freedom to run in exactly the circumstances that suit us best. Personally, I'm not a great runner and so the advantage of a treadmill for me is that I can stop whenever I want and I am no further from home than when I started. When the pavements are icy and dog walks are restricted, the treadmill provides a great space for me to get some brisk walking done, and I enjoy that feeling of pounding the pseudo-pavement.

If you prefer running outdoors then you only need to

switch to treadmills when the weather necessitates. It is a micro-adjustment to see you through some of the season and means that you can continue to exercise and maintain the fitness that will see you back outdoors as soon as the weather allows.

If the gym doesn't appeal to you, then you can change your routine and try different exercises at home. It doesn't need to be structured or boring. You can find all sorts of free workouts online, or perhaps you could put on your favourite playlist and bust some moves in the privacy of your own home. Maybe no one needs to see you put your hands in the air to Darude's 'Sandstorm' (one for the over-40s there!). The key is to get started. The biggest seasonal shake-up to my own routine is HIIT training. I am easily bored and the constant swapping of exercises, plus knowing I don't have to do them for very long, suits me down to the ground. In summer, I am able to motivate myself and complete my own training routines, but in winter I love classes where someone else has done the thinking and the planning and all I have to do is what I'm told.

Another movement to consider incorporating into your seasonal routine is yoga. Yoga is a beautiful stretch for the body and aligns with winter energy, as it allows for slower, more intentional movements, done with purpose and clarity. The winter chill can feel restrictive and yoga is a wonderful way to open up and unfurl our bodies. Yoga is accessible to all because all you need is an area to stretch, and there are so many varieties and different options for everyone. You can do a practice on a yoga mat in the full gear if you want, or you can do yoga sat in a chair at your desk, or even in bed before getting up for the day. Gently stretching our way into the day can be a gorgeous wake-up signal to the body, leaving us ready to greet the day ahead with a mellow warming energy.

The mental health benefits are huge too. Research shows that alongside enhancing muscular strength and flexibility, yogic practices reduce stress, anxiety, depression and chronic pain. Clinically, I have used specialist yoga practices to support those impacted by trauma and acute anxiety. Yoga has also been shown to improve sleep patterns and enhance overall wellbeing and quality of life. Embracing better mental health practices in a season when we are restoring and planning for the year ahead feels as though we are setting ourselves up for success. Forget what you think you know about yoga. It's not all Lycra and headstands. It is about improving your vagal tone, meaning you have lower blood pressure and better emotional regulation, as well as your heart rate variability, which in turn will lead you to better manage everyday stress and make decisions with increased clarity and certainty. Isn't that exactly what we need heading into a new season with ambitions and plans for our upcoming spring? We can access yoga anywhere, with thousands of videos available freely on streaming platforms such as YouTube, and we can even do it in our pyjamas if we want. That makes it a winter winner.

All exercise is proven to improve quality of restful and restorative sleep and it's really important that we don't see winter as a reason to stop. Remember, this is a season of supporting yourself and listening to your body. There are days when you need to rest, but maintaining movement in your routine is going to support your physical and mental health and help you get the most out of the season.

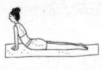 **Activity: What movement can you bring into your day?**

Consider your movement through winter. What changes do you need to make as part of your seasonal adaptation? How can you continue to move and where do you need to make changes?

If you're new to regular exercise, then what appeals? What looks fun to you? What is one small type of movement you could do today to help you build your new winter routine?

Remove any friction. What do you need in order to make exercise that little bit easier? Perhaps having cold-weather gear to hand, such as a thermal layer, a close-fitting hat, some gloves or ear muffs can go a long way to making getting outside for that walk more appealing. Even exercise at home is easier when we have warm and supportive clothes to move in. Consider what could be a blocker to you getting started and what could make you more comfortable.

Plan it. Review your diary, plan your exercise and book it in, then protect it as you would a medical appointment. It's easy to get put off or to cancel exercise but if you have a good routine in place, then you are more primed towards getting it done. Remember, it doesn't need to be rigid or boring; you could dance whilst the kettle boils for your first cuppa in the morning. Every little counts and you're more likely to move when you have a clear plan of when and where you will do so.

Remember to regularly review your routine and continue to try new activities as you move through the season. Reviewing your routine allows you to check if it's working for you, and if it's not, to change it. There is a big difference between quitting exercise altogether and quitting something you're not enjoying, so don't be afraid to try new activities. Regular reviews also prevent you feeling bored and stuck in a rut. Whatever helps you move is what works for you, so find it and enjoy it.

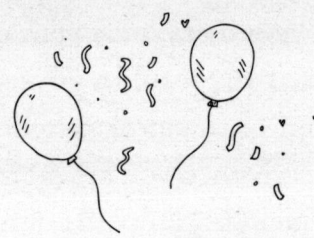

Chapter 12:
Learning to love and celebrate in winter

Sometimes a passing comment or casual conversation changes our whole approach. One such conversation happened for me when I was speaking to a colleague who had been feeling low in mood and, in her own words, 'a bit blah'. When I asked her if she had anything in the diary that she was looking forward to, she shrugged and said, 'It'll be Easter soon.' This would have been fine, except it was January! There wasn't a single point of celebration in her calendar between Christmas and Easter, meaning her next point of focus was nearly four months away and in another season altogether. I wrote about this for an article[1] and the response I got overwhelmingly showed that my colleague was not alone. Many people recognized that they too were leaving their calendars bare during winter and it was impacting their mood.

It got me thinking about some of our struggles with winter and whether this lack of socializing was compounding a feeling of a never-ending winter and a collective dip in mood. There isn't much in the collective calendar once the festive season and New Year's Eve have passed, which means we need to introduce the points of love and celebration ourselves. We cannot keep empty calendars but expect our hearts to be full of connection. Soulful celebration of love both for and in winter is an essential. We need to find our own way of marking the passing of time, in order to prevent feelings of a joyless void stretching endlessly. We can include so much to look forward to in winter, but we have to plan for it and make it extra special in order to shake off that listless feel to the start of the year.

Creating a (right kind of) busy calendar

I first started celebrating Chinese New Year in 2023. It was the year of the Water Rabbit, which is deemed a symbol of longevity, peace and prosperity in Chinese culture. When researching articles about the Lunar New Year, one line repeatedly stood out to me: '2023 is predicted to be a year of hope.' Given the cost-of-living crisis, the war in Ukraine and the fact that we were emerging blinking into the daylight after the darkness of the pandemic, a year of hope felt like something worth celebrating. I was drawn to this celebration and shared this research on a WhatsApp group. My friend Odelia immediately replied, 'Thank goodness for that! We need hope!' That was exactly how I felt.

I celebrated in a fairly small way. I made rabbit-shaped cookies and shared them with neighbours. I messaged people on the day and wished them a happy and prosperous new year. I took some time to read and learn more about the meaning behind the celebrations and I watched some traditional lion and dragon dances streaming across YouTube. It was a small celebration but it happened on 22 January and it provided a point of celebration and love in a month when the calendar was otherwise blank.

Ever since then, I have started to deliberately book things in January, February and March. I particularly like booking comedy gigs; there is something extra special about being huddled in a venue with other people all determined to have a laugh. There is a solidarity that says, 'Look at us, out and about, when it's cold and dark and we could be at home.' Whereas December can feel a crush of pressure and social obligation, January through March offers a sense of space for more deliberate and less hasty connection. I have more space for spontaneity and have learned to say yes more at the start of the calendar year, and it makes the time pass quickly, accelerated by fun and novelty.

In recent years, there has been a rise in popularity of people claiming that January is far too long. There is no logical explanation for this, as January has the same 31 days it's always had, yet it has become really popular to send memes stating 'It's 72 January today' or bemoaning that January is never-ending. However, this isn't the experience of a varied January. If we have different points of connection in the diary, see different people, have different conversations, then that variety offers a sense of time which isn't just a seamless blur. Often a slightly earlier payday ahead of the Christmas break means that financially January can feel very stretched out, but of course we can predict when this will happen and counter against it as part of our winter preparation. Also, points of celebration in winter don't have to be expensive. A cuppa with a friend, a wintery walk, a home-cooked meal. Nothing needs to be pricey or strenuous on either energy or bank balance, but simply being together, to celebrate a connection, a friendship, an event or even just a random Tuesday evening, can make all the difference to a calendar that would otherwise only offer a blank page.

Choosing celebration in winter leaves us more fulfilled. Each day has more purpose, more reason, more to offer. Winter *can* be barren, but only if we make it that way. I used to keep winter bare. I didn't book, plan or organize. I ignored the cues, both from outside in nature and from within my own brain, prompting me to connect and make plans, then wondered why winter felt so empty.

If, like me, you struggle with SAD, then spending time with people is even more important. What people don't realize about depression is that our brains want to socialize. When we feel low, our brains crave connection with our clan, we want to experience love and support and physically we need the oxytocin that comes from closeness and physical contact. Hugging your best friend really can be the best therapy available to you at a point of low mood. Although our brains tell us to be social, society tells us to socially withdraw. No one wants to be the downer on a night out and we tell ourselves that we will spoil it for others. But here's the thing. There is no social contract that says you have to present as happy. You are allowed to be present in your mood state, whatever that may be. Spending time with people whom you trust and value will give you a near-instant mood boost, which makes socializing even more important in winter if you struggle with low mood. With careful planning, winter can be a season when we can utilize group energy. No one individual has to carry the responsibility for the mood; collectively we can support and help each other and build a stronger bond. Winter can feel such an isolating and lonely season if we allow it to be blocked by assumptions about others. Perhaps, in a carefully curated world of filters and Photoshop, we would all benefit from some authentic connection. When we are together, truly together, building and strengthening bonds, creating new connections and accepting ourselves and others exactly as we are, then we are in a season of warmth, community and love.

We are gifted an actual celebration of love right in the centre of winter, which is Valentine's Day, occurring on 14 February. As with all of these celebration days, we don't have to buy into the commercialism with grand gestures and gift-giving. But Valentine's Day, at its heart, is a celebration of love, and it can be a wonderful reminder to tell people we love them, whether romantically or otherwise.

I have had many different Valentine's Days throughout my life, ranging from celebrations with partners through to the newly coined 'Galentines' and 'Palentines' celebrations, which have been a gorgeous excuse to get together and celebrate friendship. Even if it's not on 14 February, I am so intensely grateful to the people in my life that taking a few moments to tell them that is a special point of connection.

> **Activity: Questions for reflection**
>
> How can you celebrate those you love this winter?
>
> What is one quality or characteristic about someone that you really love about them? How can you let them know that?
>
> Can you write a note, ping a message or call someone *right now* to let them know that you love them?
>
> How can you continue to celebrate those you love beyond the season?

Learning to love and celebrate ourselves

Prior to meeting my partner, I spent many Valentine's Days living and working in areas where I knew no one and didn't have anyone around me to connect with. I reframed any sadness I felt when I realized that I didn't need a romantic partner to celebrate love. Instead, I reflected on what I loved in my life at that moment and how I wanted to generate more love for others and myself. I reflected on what I loved about my work and took some time to acknowledge successes. I realized that sometimes we can be so focused on finding someone else to love that we completely neglect to love ourselves. We are the person who is always with us, who carries us through every situation, who never leaves us. That person deserves celebrating.

Whilst we are focusing our time and energy on love and celebration and our connection with others, winter is the perfect season to love and celebrate ourselves. We can often disconnect from ourselves in winter, distracted by festivities and then harshly critical as we judge our bodies in the face of new year, new me 'improvements'. Even the eschewing of New Year's resolutions can be problematic, as we are encouraged to 'accept our flaws' and 'accept ourselves as we are' in a way that implies we are problematically riddled with issues, and we just need to make our peace with them. What if this isn't the case? What if instead of merely accepting ourselves, we are able to celebrate ourselves? If you are British and reading this then you may be overwhelmed with a sense of awkwardness right now. We, along with many nations and cultures around the world, are not encouraged to be our own cheerleaders. We confuse confidence and self-love with arrogance and indulgence. But we shouldn't.

Celebrating ourselves is highlighting what makes us *us*. It's an acknowledgement of our individualism, our strengths, our vulnerabilities, our own philosophies and beliefs. It moves us beyond acceptance and a sense of resignation about who we are towards glorious, riotous jubilation. It's self-acceptance on steroids. It's paying attention to who we really are and learning to love and celebrate the qualities which make us special and whole. It's easy to ignore certain parts of ourselves, often the parts that we wish weren't there. The parts we don't want to carry with us. We deny so many parts of ourselves because we don't deem them good enough. Enough for whom? Society? Our families? Ourselves?

Winter is the perfect season for self-love and celebration. After all, many would deem winter as falling short and needing resigned acceptance but those of us who have embraced it know differently. What makes us whole is the sum of our parts, not just the shiny outer layer that we may present to the world. Learning to not only love but to actively celebrate those parts of us which may stay hidden from others brings a level of self-acceptance that lays the foundational stones of self-confidence. What a glorious gift to celebrate yourself, all of yourself, and to start your year with self-love and confidence as your foundations.

We can utilize our reflective winter mood to pay more attention to ourselves. It is possible that the busier 'doing' seasons have swept us along and we haven't paused for breath to really understand where we are and how we are doing. We have lost the art of checking in on ourselves. We are so busy, so distracted, so connected to external stimuli that we have lost the simple art of tuning in and gently questioning ourselves. Are we where we want to be? Are we happy with how we got here? Are we following a path that suits us best? Alongside these broader questions, we can be more specific. When was the last time I celebrated myself? When did I last show myself some love and encouragement? Winter reflection allows us the headspace and opportunity to really connect with and celebrate our true selves.

Personally, I find winter is when I can best celebrate my ambivert status. I've never really connected with the idea of being wholly introvert or wholly extrovert and I used to struggle with that. We seem to celebrate extroverts in society and consider them the more fun and gregarious among us, whilst having some sympathy for the quiet introvert who never wants to leave their house. There doesn't seem to be a space for those who are somewhere in-between, the ambiverts, yet I think this is by far the most common state.

For many of us, our response will be situation-dependent. I know that I can absolutely show up and be front and centre when needed but then take several days recharging my energy to recover. For me it's a balance, and winter is a time when I can celebrate that. I can be present in festivities but also recharge my energy, by getting cosy in my winter retreat and indulging in some gentler activities which rekindle my inner glow before that light dims or burns out. It's a season that doesn't make me feel weird for not being one thing or the other. There is space for all emotions and all emotional states in winter and it's a great opportunity to rediscover and celebrate everything that makes us who we are.

Self-love and self-celebration can take many forms. There is something particularly important about taking care of your physical body as an act of self-love and kindness. When we take care of ourselves physically, we are sending a message. We remind ourselves that we are worthy of love and that we are worthy of expending energy on self-care. This isn't about appearance or needing to look a certain way; rather, this is about identifying an act of self-care that will benefit you and ensuring that you make time for it.

For example, when the central heating and colder weather can leave our skin dehydrated and dry, there is kindness in applying a layer of moisturiser to soothe and prevent cracked skin. We can just grab a blob of hand cream on the move, quickly rubbing it in whilst on our way to do something else. Or we could pause for a moment of mindfulness and recognize this act of self-love. We can view our skin through the lens of gratitude for its hard work and the protection it offers us. We can thank our skin. A moment like this is not big, it's not expensive, but it is deliberate and mindful. It is self-love in action and on purpose. It matters.

 **Activity: Getting started with self-celebration**

Take some time for reflection. Make your favourite drink, in your favourite mug, and retreat to your cosy winter space with a notebook to jot down some thoughts.

Reflect on the questions below and make a note of anything that comes up for you, then use it to build your self-celebration plan:

1) What would it mean if I were to celebrate myself? How would I feel? How would I know I was celebrating myself?
2) What is something about myself that I have forgotten to celebrate or love recently?
3) What do I feel is not worth celebrating and how can I choose to love and honour that part of me?
4) Which part of me do I tend to ignore? How can I highlight that part of myself and show it some love?
5) What is a small celebratory activity that I can do right now to show myself unconditional love and radical self-acceptance?

We can be our own worst critics at times and if the concept of self-love and celebration is new, then it takes some practice to adopt the mindset. That's OK, we have a whole season to adapt and build a self-love practice. The important part is realizing that there is space for *all* of us in winter. We don't need to pretend to be anything other than exactly what we are. What a glorious space that is to spend the season in. A space of love, acknowledgement and authenticity. When we experience the slow-down and the hush, we have the time to spend with ourselves, reconnecting and getting to know ourselves again. That is definitely worth celebrating.

Celebrating winter itself

As well as celebrating *in* winter, I love to celebrate the arrival of winter itself. I imagine winter arriving at the party of our year and immediately feeling unwelcome as it hears those around us mutter, 'Ugh, I hate winter.' I like to turn that on its head and hold a celebration specifically to welcome winter with open arms.

Given winter solstice happens just before Christmas, it isn't often an occasion that I invite others to, as people tend to be getting ready to travel or jump right into the Christmas chaos and so it can be overwhelming to add something else to their already squeezed diaries. However, I secretly revel in the time to celebrate, just me and winter. I feel as though I am welcoming and warmly embracing an old friend. My welcome to winter has become an annual ritual and I really encourage you to build your own.

Celebrating winter – a ritual

My ritual is what works well for me but is by no means the only way to welcome winter. As we explored earlier (see page 129), there are many established celebrations and festivals that you can join in with if you don't already, but I also encourage you to create your own ritual to welcome winter into your home and your heart.

My ritual takes place on winter solstice and varies in location depending on where I am working and what is happening in my life at the time. My favourite space is my cosy winter retreat at home, but I have also welcomed winter during a walk and even in a busy city centre, beneath the impressive display of Christmas lights.

As with many festivals, light plays a part in my ritual. If at home, I light a candle; if out and about, then anywhere where I can connect with winter light works well. Taking some time to settle and pause, I reflect on the following questions, and I encourage you to do the same:

1. What is the light, no matter how small, that I can celebrate this winter?
2. What provides a glimmer, a guiding light or a gentle reflection of goodness back into any darkness?
3. What lit my path this year and what will I light in preparation for next year?

We know that winter carries more light into our year, offering us a gentle illumination throughout the first three months. It is the soft launch of the year ahead and it is a time that gently reveals what we need, what we want, what we focus on and what we have. This ritual turns the page and reveals a new seasonal chapter. It begins our reflection and provides a moment of grounding at a point of the year that can feel very chaotic. I welcome winter and it welcomes all of us. When we open our arms to winter, we truly feel its embrace.

Chapter 13:
A calm(er) Christmas

In an increasingly secular world, you could be forgiven for thinking that you could avoid or bow out of a Christian religious festival. However, despite just 46.2% of the UK identifying as Christian,[1] with 'no religion' being the next highest category (37.2%), Christmas remains ubiquitous with celebration and tradition in winter.

When I was younger, I was astounded by how many non-Christians got their tinsel in a tangle and felt so much stress during the weeks before Christmas. I didn't understand why people who didn't *have* to celebrate were going ahead with something that clearly brought them no joy. As I got older, I began to recognize the social significance of Christmas and the wider role it plays, not just societally but commercially. I also began to understand how winter itself can provide the perfect antidote to the pressures of Christmas.

Many of us who follow a different religion, or indeed no religion at all, will still find ourselves celebrating Christmas.

It can be a wonderful, fun, joy-filled affair and I don't want to paint a negative picture. However, for many, Christmas can bring uncomfortable family dynamics to the surface and other challenges which need to be managed. Although I write about Christmas here, the advice shared can be applied to any festival, celebration or family event. This is not a 'survival guide' for Christmas, but rather an understanding of how winter itself can support us through this potentially chaotic start to the season.

Growing up, Christmas in my house was never optional. I have a Catholic dad and a Protestant mum and that made Christmas a big deal. Christian faith aside, my mum was the real reason why Christmas was such a focal point in our house. My mum *loved* Christmas when we were little. She'd get super-excited about everything. The tree would have a colour theme for the decorations and any wrapping paper that didn't fit the aesthetic saw the present promptly hidden around the back. We'd stock the house full of food, with the best items stored safely out of reach of smaller hands. Mum and Dad would dedicate an evening, with the radio on and a glass of wine apiece, to write their Christmas cards to friends and family, commenting out loud on who had moved where and prompting each other on the names of friends' children.

One of my earliest Christmas memories is of being in the trolley in my pyjamas as Mum and I got up at silly o'clock and went to do the BIG Christmas shop. This was when the internet and online shopping were a mere glint in a developer's eye and so you had to go and do battle in person. With list and trolley at the ready, you'd spend the entire shop double-checking that you hadn't forgotten anything, as the shops would be shut on Christmas Day and you hadn't a hope of getting your mitts on anything accidentally missed off.

As a child, all this excitement and gentle chaos was fun, but as an adult, the other side of Christmas soon became apparent. I was able to see that the same celebration could be both gorgeous and troublesome in equal parts. What is fun to witness as a child can be incredibly stressful to manage as an adult. Again, I became aware that there could be a better way to manage Christmas, using the gentle energy of winter to support us. I have realigned my own Christmases with winter and it's an approach I recommend you try too.

One of the pressures of Christmas is the pressure to create traditions. This seems to be particularly prevalent when we have children and we feel a need to create our own family traditions, which we repeat year after year. Whilst holding a beautiful intention, I believe traditions can add a very unnatural annual pressure and set us up for future stress and sadness.

I accidentally started the family tradition of my maternal grandparents always spending Christmas with us. I didn't mean to; I simply wasn't being listened to. I was quite a quiet child with a far noisier sibling. I asked Mum and Dad several times whether my grandparents were coming to ours for Christmas Day. I kept being ignored as my sister diverted the attention back to her. So I wrote to my grandparents and asked them directly. In my defence, I regularly wrote to my grandparents and so it felt very natural for me to write and ask them if they were spending Christmas with us. My grandparents, upon receiving such a question, saw a sweet invitation masked in a child's letter and they promptly phoned my mum to accept.

The first I knew about the mix-up was that there was a lot of commotion in the hallway, as everyone stood around the landline where my mum had just replaced the receiver. My sister turned to me as I walked downstairs to investigate the fuss and said, 'Ooh, who else have you invited, Steph? The Queen??' and Mum and Dad began talking very loudly and opening the wine. My protestations that I hadn't asked them *to* Christmas, I had asked *if* they were coming for Christmas, fell on deaf ears and I was teased about my slip-up for years to come.

Whilst it may have caused a bit of upheaval and extra planning for my parents, I confess that I regret nothing. Having my grandparents around me that year was one of the best Christmas presents I could have asked for and their Christmas visits became a regular part of our festivities. My accidental invite created countless memories for years to come and I am intensely grateful that I got to celebrate so many Christmases with them both.

The problem with this tradition only revealed itself over time. Everything felt wrong, really wrong, when my grandparents weren't here any more to celebrate with us. Everything from raising a glass to saying the toast over dinner and deciding who sat where suddenly felt different, missing and off. It created an unbearable sadness. Misslieness, the feeling of loneliness caused by the absence of someone who is usually around, stings just a little more during celebratory occasions. It's not just those who have died, it's also those we want to be with but who cannot be there to celebrate with us. Divorced parents missing their children, those who work away from home, or those too far in either physical or emotional distance to be with. Wanting someone to be there and feeling their absence can leave us with an ache in our hearts that no amount of jollity can shift.

There is something to be said about the pressure of traditions and whether our endless pursuit of the 'traditional' Christmas, creating a legacy for our children to shoulder, is actually making us happy. Doing anything with the expectation of doing it for ever adds a pressure. On our Christmas Day dog walks, we always bump into more people than usual. Some are very chipper and jolly and call out 'Merry Christmas', typically whilst walking a dachshund wearing a dinky yet jaunty Fair Isle sweater (you've got a visual). Others barely raise a smile and are clearly enduring, not enjoying, their Christmas constitutional. I quietly asked some of the grumpier gang why they were out walking and the words 'family tradition' were darkly muttered. Not much Christmas cheer to be had there. Are we right to keep pushing traditions, even when they don't work for everyone? When situations change, maybe we should change with them. Maybe the celebration we set up doesn't *need* to be for ever. Maybe there is a better way.

Does Christmas have a right to be forgotten?

There is a wonderful French concept called *le droit à l'oubli* or 'the right to be forgotten'. This concept has nothing to do with Christmas or celebrations; it's the common name for a legal right that was first established in May 2014 in the European Union. The European Court of Justice ruled that European data protection laws gave individuals the right to ask search engines to delist certain results. In other words, individuals had a right to be forgotten by search engines and for certain results to be removed or no longer associated with searches of their name.

I think Christmas should have its own *droit à l'oubli*. We should be able to wipe the slate clean every Christmas and review it afresh. We can appreciate what's gone before and then approach it as a new season, a new phase, a new celebration. Rather than crash into it, stressing about how to deliver what we feel is expected of us, we can start by stopping. We can sit down and ask ourselves, 'What do I need this year?'

Although the date of Christmas doesn't shift, our mood, energy and desires will vary from year to year, and we need to pay attention to that. Some of our traditions won't serve us as well as they have in previous years and that's OK. We don't have to forget them altogether, but we can decide afresh what it is that we want to include and build our celebration around our wants and needs. Before we begin any planning with others, we need to know what it is that *we* need from the celebrations. We need to give ourselves and others permission to start again. So many of us feel stuck in a rigid 'traditional' format but often this rigidity stops serving any useful purpose and becomes constraining and uncomfortable. We have more fluidity and choice than we realize, but it means managing and deconstructing that which has been built before.

Some years we may be all for the chaos and the socializing and the whirlwind. Other years, we may need a quieter and gentler celebration. Some years we may need to not celebrate at all. Trying to copy and paste Christmas onto different years, moods, energies and environments only sets us up for friction and failure.

We can utilize our winter reflection to immediately align the festivities we want to follow with the energy of winter. Christmas can offer a gentler, kinder and more authentic start to the festive period and lead us into a happier and healthier season.

The stories we tell

We can get so caught up in the expectations of others that we forget to check in on ourselves to see where we are and what we need right now. We need to let go of this idea that we *have* to celebrate Christmas in a certain way, or that we *have* to celebrate it at all. Winter is a time for sharing stories but we need to be careful about the stories we tell ourselves, the reactions we pre-empt and the obligations we create.

My father-in-law loves spending Christmas Day alone.

The story I used to tell myself about this was that it was awful for him to be alone and so we used to force ourselves on him, arriving laden with gifts and hugs and general Christmas overbearance. However, when we had an open discussion about it, I realized that not only would he be absolutely fine if he didn't see us, he preferred not to. For him, Christmas and his Christmas routine are a solo ritual and he wants to spend the day alone. There is no sadness for him in his Christmas story and I needed to rescript it to make sure that there was no sadness in mine. He's not interested in his incessantly nagging daughter-in-law (waves!) tentatively asking him about his diabetes and whether he needs to measure his blood sugar again as he opens a second box of chocolates. He wants to be left alone and there is nothing sad about that. It's a conversation we revisit every year, as we want to check his plans still work for him, but, for now, he finds being alone joyful, and we do see him on the surrounding days, just not on the day itself. It's really important to let go of assumptions and reflect year on year about what we all need and want and to allow others to own their stories.

Some of the lengths we go to in order to achieve the Christmas we want are astonishing. One year, my oldest friend and I caught up ahead of Christmas and when I asked her what she was doing, she replied:

'I'm going to tell my cousin Francesca I'm at Mum and Dad's, and tell Mum and Dad I'm with Francesca, and then tell Steven (boyfriend) I'm with you, but actually I'm going to spend the

day in bed, on my own, with a box of chocolates, a movie, a glass of wine and do exactly what I want to do for a change. Bliss.'

I was struck by how, in order to do what she wanted, she was having to lie to everyone who cares about her and loves her. The very people who would want to see her relaxed and happy. Maybe the idea of doing exactly what we want isn't selfish but eminently sensible and we need to be open about that.

By understanding our own Christmas story, we can spot where we clash with others. If your mum wants everyone gathered together for a huge noisy lunch but you want to spend the day curled up with a book and your favourite snacks, then you can immediately see the clash and begin to articulate what you need. Remember, no one has a right to your time, space and energy. Only you have that right. We cannot control other people, or make them behave differently. The only control we have is over ourselves and our behaviours. The only story we can tell is our own.

How we want to spend our day and our celebration should not be cemented in traditions that suited us one year, possibly in completely different circumstances, mood and health states. Instead, we may be happier with fresh plans. Communication over assumptions. Pause over pressure.

> **Activity: Reshaping your Christmas**
>
> Ask yourself the following five questions:
>
> 1) If you picture exactly what *you* would want this Christmas, what are you seeing?
> 2) How do you want to feel at the end of the Christmas period?
> 3) What is the story you tell yourself about your celebration?
> 4) How can you challenge or change that story this year to fit with your energy and desires?
> 5) Which part of your past Christmases do you think has a right to be forgotten?

Managing the expectations of others

Often the pressure we feel doesn't come from within but from others. Navigating the Christmas timetable can feel as though it is a lesson in diplomacy and delicate negotiation. We can witness behaviour akin to bullying and emotional blackmail, which no one puts on their Christmas wish list.

It is really useful to have open conversations with family early, so that everyone has a chance to contribute their thoughts, ideas and preferences, and these can be discussed together, without any additional timeline pressure. Also, if someone in your circle has made assumptions, then there is time to correct these and make alternative plans.

We sometimes avoid discussions about celebrations because they feel emotionally laden and so they quickly get assigned to the 'too difficult' pile. Of course, some celebrations are gorgeous and happy occasions and I certainly don't want to suggest that all of them are fraught with difficulty. But for the 1 in 3 of us who is apathetic about or actively dislikes Christmas,[2] other people are often the root cause of the way we feel and it's important to recognize this in order to identify what needs to change.

If you have a family member who demands your time and energy over Christmas, it can feel hard to say no. But you are allowed to. You are also allowed to do things differently to accommodate your needs. You are allowed to write your own Christmas story.

I recommend the following approaches to managing these conversations with others:

1. **Find the shared values.** If everyone seems to want different outcomes for the same day, then try to find the common ground. Forget focusing on venues and timetables and instead highlight what is shared. Maybe it's everyone getting together, sharing a meal, opening gifts or seeing children. Whatever it is, common ground is easier to navigate, so start there and build your plans.

2. **Be honest about the challenges.** If you have clashes, make them everyone's problem to solve, rather than just your own. Many of us are geographically spread around, and trying to see everyone by traversing motorways up and down the country is not exactly relaxing in what can be a few precious days off. I've often joked that I've gone back to work for a rest! Rather than exhaust yourself by trying to accommodate everyone, share the problems and challenges and find group solutions, recognizing where compromise is needed. It's easier to highlight challenges when everyone can see them.

3. **Use the 'broken record' technique.** The broken record technique sees us repeat the same message over and over until the other person hears us. If you say to someone, 'We are staying home just us this year,' then whatever response or challenge you face, you simply repeat that. If they reply, 'Oh but that's not fair, we really wanted to see you. We wanted to be together,' then you simply reply, 'I understand that, but we are staying home just us this year.' This approach saves you energy and prevents you becoming entangled in arguments. The more you repeat, the stronger the message becomes and once you prove that you will not be emotionally blackmailed or coerced into changing your plans, then it actually becomes easier to discuss. No matter

what someone says, or accuses you of, simply repeat yourself. It's not confrontational, but it is confident, and it's then easier to arrange alternative plans, if you wish to.

4. **Find an alternative date.** One of the biggest challenges with Christmas is trying to get everyone together at the same time on the same day. I really recommend spreading the celebrations and having a get-together ahead of the day itself. This alleviates so many pressures: the traffic, the shops being closed, the weather causing disruptions. This also means that, if you have been unable to avoid plans you would rather not be attending, then you are free to celebrate your own Christmas however you want to. Present alternative dates to your circle and wish each other a Merry (almost!) Christmas.

Fluctuating needs and support

Just as the energy of the seasons ebbs and flows, so will our need for help and support. Sometimes I like it when people do nothing to help. When I want to crack on with cooking, getting everyone out of the kitchen and out of my way can be a reprieve. Although I like socializing, these snatched moments of peace keep my social batteries topped up. However, at other times I can really resent the lack of support and wish that people would step up to help me. This will entirely depend on my energy levels and subsequent mood and this is why it is so important to tune in and not make assumptions or have expectations of ourselves. When we know what we need, it is far easier to ask for support and, most importantly, be specific about the kind of help we need.

My friend Georgina shared that a few of her old school friends got together one year to have an early Christmas celebration. Not wanting any one person to feel the burden of catering, they'd all agreed to prepare and bring a dish. One of the group was tasked with bringing the red cabbage. I don't know if this is a uniquely British dish, but if you've never had it, it's a side dish prepared by cooking red cabbage with cider vinegar, wine, sugar, cinnamon sticks, star anise and vegetable stock until the cabbage is tender. The flavours are delicious and it provides a sweet acidity to the meal.

The friend who was asked to bring the red cabbage responded, 'No problem!' and everyone went away to prepare their dishes accordingly. Imagine the surprise when, on the day, this particular friend arrived brandishing . . . a red cabbage. As in a whole, raw, red cabbage. No prep. No effort. No delicious side dish. The assumption she'd made was that she'd do the shopping and the host would do the cooking because, 'I thought you loved cooking!' Lesson learned: if you are asking for help and support then be very specific about what you need from others.

No surprises

My partner despairs at the way my family and I buy presents for each other. We tell each other exactly what we want from each person. I mean *exactly*. We send photos and links. There is no element of surprise and my partner thinks it strange and transactional, but we love it.

It started when I worked for the NHS. Earning the sort of salary that a 'vocation' offers, I didn't have the money to waste on presents that people would send straight to the re-gift drawer, or worse, the rubbish bin. I texted my family one year and simply said, 'Without meaning to spoil the surprise, I would like to get you something you really want rather than guess and get it wrong, so let me know if there is something that you would really like.' Everyone immediately jumped on board and we were soon exchanging links to the exact gifts that we wished to receive. I used to stipulate that it was something that people *wanted* rather than needed, a real treat, but I've since changed my mind. When you have just moved house, or retired, or have been through a life event, sometimes someone buying you something you need can provide some very real help and support; that is a gift in itself.

Even though I know exactly what I will be getting from someone in my family, it doesn't lessen the gift in any way. It brings anticipatory joy, which heightens the experience. If you can ask people what they would like and, even better, set an agreed and affordable budget, then you are saving everyone time, money and energy.

Outside of my own immediate family, all my adult in-laws don't buy each other presents at all. Instead, we spend the money on a meal out together in January. I had noticed that presents were becoming increasingly more generic and expensive as we compensated for a lack of time and connection by throwing a credit card at the problem. Although I always remain very grateful for any presents received, I was painfully aware that we were buying each other 'stuff' and actually our favourite part of Christmas was catching up and spending time together. Recognizing that we didn't need to spend money buying each other yet more scarves and scented candles (we only possess one neck each and can only burn so many candles before our homes turn into a fire hazard), we use that meal together as an investment in our relationships. It feels a far better way to spend our money, and also gives us something to look forward to post-Christmas.

You can't buy a perfect Christmas

Money can be a blocker to connection, particularly when we are trying to avoid uncomfortable emotions. We put our money in place of our time, or to try to repair or gloss over a challenging or ruptured relationship with a gift. Perhaps we are aware that we haven't kept in touch with someone, or perhaps we are looking to compensate for or mask challenging feelings.

Recognizing that you cannot buy a united emotional response at Christmas can be powerful, liberating and save you a small fortune.

Although we can feel uncomfortable having conversations about money, people are often intensely grateful when we raise the issue and give them permission to do things differently, in a way that suits them and their budget. This is particularly true in families and social circles where incomes, budgets and expenditure differ. Talking money can feel as though we are committing the ultimate social faux pas but there is a financial reality to celebration and 1 in 4 of us will struggle to afford Christmas,[3] a number that is only increasing. It may feel uncomfortable because it isn't a conversation we have every day but it is OK to have an open and frank discussion where you set boundaries around money.

There are many different ways to manage the issue. Perhaps you agree a secret Santa where every person only buys one present and you agree a maximum spend. You could agree a theme to your gift to make it more creative and fun, whilst keeping costs down. Gifting this way also alleviates a lot of stress and prevents last-minute panic-spending. Although Christmas is imbued with childlike joy, we need to have grown-up conversations about money. If you have multiple Christmas expenses, you can alleviate your own and others' financial burden, which can be the greatest gift of all.

Connecting with your community

Winter offers us the gift of gratitude and we can feel it very acutely around Christmas. When we step in from the cold and feel our extremities prinkle as we thaw out, it can make us very aware and very grateful for what we have, and more minded to give to those less fortunate.

Helping out isn't just good for others, it's also great for our brains. When we help others, we activate an area in the brain called the mesolimbic pathway. The mesolimbic pathway is a dopaminergic pathway associated with reward, which transports dopamine and engages the emotional part of the brain. Put simply, when we help others out, we activate our reward centre and are rewarded with endorphins, the feel-good factor. This process is also known as 'helper's high' and has been shown to boost self-esteem and happiness and combat feelings of depression.

The Charities Aid Foundation found that many of those they surveyed said that the festive period was a traditional time to give, but we don't need to put pressure on ourselves to build yet another tradition or feel further financial burden. Our availability in every sense will vary year on year and we can respect that. However, we can seek out small acts of giving which make a huge difference without costing a lot of money, time or energy. If you are feeling low on resources, you can still do something to support someone else and receive the very welcome brain boost, without depleting your own energy stocks.

If you have a coat that you no longer wear, there are organizations that will accept these and give them to the homeless, ensuring that people have a warm outer layer to protect them against the bitter temperatures. Often these donation points sit at large train stations, so this simple act could be completed one morning as part of your daily commute to work, costing you nothing in terms of time, money or energy, yet making a life-changing, possibly life-saving difference to someone else. If you have a little more in the tank, perhaps volunteer to collect donated coats from your colleagues or friends and make a group donation.

The Warm Welcome Space[4] initiative in the UK has seen companies sharing their physical spaces as a way to keep communities together and prevent loneliness and isolation. What started as a response to the cost-of-living crisis has seen the development of a vibrant and growing connected community. Companies and buildings of all sizes can offer a warm, safe and welcoming space to others and it costs nothing more than opening your doors.

I saw a beautiful offering from a bookshop which opened on Christmas morning for tea, warmth and mince pies. The emphasis was on the doors, not the tills, being open and the aim was to provide company and conversation for those who wanted it and who would otherwise be alone.

Food banks are always a good way to support others and often will share a list of products they need so you can donate meaningfully. Or you can buy small Christmas gifts for children in hospital or the care system, to ensure they have something to open on Christmas Day. You can donate to organizations that will provide education, tools and resources to a multitude of people who need help, in all kinds of social and challenging situations. You can find a way to support what matters most to you.

There are so many wonderful ways to spend time with people, and the sense of connection and community is inspiring. Whether you volunteer, hold an event, visit people or open your home to others, there are multiple ways to give back at Christmas, and a small amount of your time can make a huge difference to someone else. In a season of connection, feeling closer to your community can align you with winter, right from the start.

Making room for all the emotions

Christmas is an unpredictable time emotionally. In recent years, many people have reported a weight of emotion in the run-up to Christmas without knowing why. It can be no one particular 'thing', just a general heaviness that seems to hang in the air, perhaps caused by illness, financial challenges or ongoing global issues. It is important to make room for all our emotions at Christmas, not just the ones we think we should be feeling. There are no rules, and when we relax the constraints and make space for everything, we can better support ourselves and others to feel happier and healthier.

I do not want you to mistake Christmas, or indeed any celebration in winter, as something to be endured, not enjoyed. There are many sparks of joy and glimmers that can be felt throughout Christmas, but if you are balancing those with more difficult emotions then it's important to know that that's OK and very normal. Small tweaks and changes allow us to make space for all emotions and manage them accordingly.

 Activity: Dealing with all the emotions

1) Acknowledge your emotions, both to yourself and to others. Often being authentic about how we feel is enough. Acknowledging how we feel and letting others know means that we can release the pressure of wearing a mask. Being honest and saying, 'I don't feel how I expected to,' or 'I feel sad and low on energy right now,' allows you to take actions to protect and boost your health and opens you to more support and help from others.

2) Manage your inputs. If you are finding Christmas challenging, then manage what you absorb. Everything from Christmas music, to conversations, to social media can be reduced to support your mood. Pay attention to what you are tuning in to and ask yourself if it is serving you well. There is a reason why *Die Hard* is such a popular 'Christmas

film' – and that's because it has nothing to do with Christmas! It is a reprieve. Take a moment to manage your inputs and switch off anything that isn't working for you.

3) Take time out to worry. We can try to push worries and anxieties to the back of our minds at Christmas but they don't respond well to being ignored. Imagine the walls of your mind are made of elastic; the harder you try to push a thought away, the harder it will ping back at you. Instead of ignoring anything that is worrying you, make space for it in your day. Find a quiet spot where you won't be interrupted, set a timer for 15 minutes and bring to mind everything that is worrying you, and deliberately focus on it. The idea is that you give yourself permission to worry. It may not sound long, but you will be surprised how quickly your brain gets bored of worrying and wanders off track. If it does, gently guide your thoughts back to your worries. Once the timer goes off, stand up and physically shake off your worries. If any pop back into your head, tell yourself that you will focus on them at the next timed worry slot but not before. Anxiety responds very well to this boundary and it can mean that worries dominate 15 minutes of your day rather than the whole day itself. (Top tip: never use bedtime for a worry slot; you need to be able to

> physically move away from it as a cue to your brain. That's harder to do if you are in bed and then try to go to sleep, so keep any worrying out of your bedtime routine.)

The old English saying 'huck muck' describes the confusion or frustration that comes with things being out of place. Christmas brings about some strange displacement in our homes as we shift furniture around to make room for a tree and we've all experienced the irritation of trying to locate the Sellotape which we know is around here somewhere. It also brings about some strange displacement in our hearts. Feelings can be jumbled and displaced and we can lose sight of ourselves over Christmas, making it a discombobulating time.

The key to a calm(er) Christmas is to make space for it all. Acknowledge the pressures we feel, the challenges we face and the moods we experience. Taking time to assess year on year, without assumption or judgement, what will work best for you and for those you love sets you up for success. Those traditions that you love can be remembered or reinvented without the pressure. Perhaps, if you have always made the Christmas cake using your great aunt's recipe which needs to be started in August, you can make a toast to your great aunt over a slice of shop-bought cake this year. Adapt and adjust your Christmas to be whatever you need it to be. Remember, Christmas has the right to be forgotten, so wipe the slate clean, plan for what works for you and enjoy the celebration you have, even if that is no celebration at all. There is space for every kind of Christmas and every kindness at Christmas, especially to yourself. Write yourself a kinder and calmer Christmas story this year.

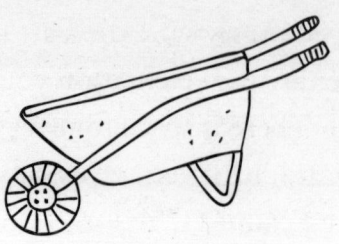

Chapter 14:
A winter garden

If nature provides an entire library of information, then our garden can act as our own personal study. It's easy to see winter as a time to close the door on our outside space. After all, as the temperature drops, we are less inclined to sit, eat or drink outside. Smaller feet are less likely to run around the garden and even our pets can sit at the back door, meowing or huffing demands that we turn the heat up and the rain down before they want to venture outside. But, as the quiet hush settles, our gardens continue to share their wisdom with us.

    I spend a lot of time in my garden in winter. Not so much actively gardening as just simply *being* in the garden. Time spent wandering first thing, hands wrapped around a warming mug, spending a few tranquil moments waking up with my garden. I like to brush my hands against the leaves of the beautifully named photinia 'Red Robin' shrub, still showing up brightly, offering vivid splashes of red and green. I spend time contemplating the buds now evident, envisioning their future tucked into those tiny pods of potential. I wonder about their plans for the spring as I consider my own.

I like that there is less to do in the garden. Unlike the rooms in our homes that don't offer a seasonal slow-down, when walking around our gardens in winter, we are not confronted with a huge to-do list. Leaves aren't demanding to be cleared, plants aren't reaching out, imploring us to trim them. All is calm and seemingly still, yet gently growing, stretching and unfurling into the season as we prepare for spring.

I'm not a great gardener. I love the aesthetic of a beautiful garden but lack the space, time and talent to achieve it. I am resigned to accepting and appreciating what is already in my garden and I do my best to support and look after it. It is a very low-key but much-loved extension of my home. Simply taking time out with a cup of tea allows a much-needed tune-in to an area I really know nothing about. I only have a dinky garden and feel continually amazed that my tiny space holds an enormous Californian lilac, a showy shrub that I am in love with. It blooms twice a year and the periwinkle blue flowers provide an astonishing centrepiece in an otherwise fairly bland space.

Seeing it apparently overgrown, I was on the cusp of cutting it right back to 'save it' and prevent any damage occurring, but my regular morning observations showed me that it was a safe haven for the sparrows, wrens and robins that visited it. It wasn't that they were nesting in there, but they seemed very content to hang out there. They came together several times per day, their loud gossipy chirruping stealing my attention and drawing my gaze outside through the window. I realized that this shrub was a metaphorical camp fire for these birds and I didn't want to take that away from them. They, too, needed to come together in winter to share their year, plan for the next and tell stories. I appreciate this might sound fanciful, but had I not spent time outside in the mornings, I wouldn't have noticed this feathered convention and would have taken up the shears with gusto. Instead, I learned how to support the branches and gently prune the very edges to encourage growth (much like a trim at the hairdressers), and otherwise left it well alone.

If you don't have access to a garden of your own, then winter is a great time to explore local green spaces and parks. There is a different energy in the air; a solidness to the atmosphere; a grounding and reassuring sense of peace providing a comforting tranquillity. The popular Japanese activity of *shinrin-yoku*, or forest bathing, has been proven to have many different health benefits, including reduced blood pressure, lowered cortisol and improved memory and concentration, as well as enhanced overall wellbeing.[1]

Being amongst trees provides us with a broader sense of perspective. There is something reassuring about standing amongst that which was likely here long before us and will continue to stand long after us. We can sense the strength of the root network beneath our feet, and that gentle pulse of winter energy is louder and clearer when communicated through trees and plants. We often find big emotions visit, but don't overwhelm, when we stand amongst these giants.

If there isn't a woodland or forest nearby for you to explore, you can still gain many health benefits by connecting with nature in a park or walking along a leafy street, or you can move your garden indoors with houseplants or growing herbs on windowsills. The benefits of gardening are well documented, no matter how you engage with it. Children who engage with nature have been shown to benefit from better social relationships, family connections and emotional and mental wellbeing.[2] Gardening has been shown to moderate stress, reduce depression and anxiety and improve cognitive and educational outcomes for children and adolescents.[3] Children also benefit from the sense of achievement and mastery that comes with growing things and it can offer satisfaction and empowerment, particularly for those children who may not thrive within the confines of traditional academic settings. If your child isn't excelling inside the classroom, it may well be that they will thrive outside of it.

Urban gardening utilizes the balconies and rooftops of city spaces to encourage us to develop green fingers at any age and in any location. Troughs are popping up everywhere from train stations to outside city hospitals to try to bring the benefits of greenery and nature to all. These spaces are sorely needed, as nearly 10 million of us living in the UK reside in neighbourhoods without access to green spaces such as parks or nature trails. However, we can all benefit from gardening, even on a small scale. Growing a pot of herbs or keeping a houseplant has been shown to offer mental health benefits, and these benefits grow as we do. Adults who garden feel greater life satisfaction, quality of life, improved energy levels and enjoy notable reductions in stress, anger, depression, anxiety and fatigue.[4]

Thankfully for me, the positive impacts of gardening are not linked to skill level. Even five minutes pottering with plants has been shown to improve self-esteem and mood.[5] You don't need to be aiming for an award-winning space; a brief connection with nature is enough, especially in winter when we welcome the extra mood boost.

If this doesn't feel like 'proper' gardening, don't underestimate the power of nature. Research shows that even looking at pictures of the countryside and surrounding nature has been associated with reduced pain, increased productivity and greater overall life satisfaction.[6] However you engage with nature, green spaces and gardens, it all counts.

Learning from nature

Our gardens teach us valuable lessons on how to behave in winter, lessons which are applicable beyond our green spaces and into our wider lives.

One of my favourite winter gardening tips is to leave your perennials alone.[7] Perennials are those plants in our gardens that return year after year and we need to resist being too tidy with them. Leaving the dry leaves and stems on your herbaceous perennials (those that die back in autumn/winter and rebloom in spring), will provide a safe shelter for many insects to move into over winter and these plants will return again and again without intervention.

This is a reminder that winter isn't a time for radical overhaul. Now isn't the time to start aggressively pruning or hacking away at a habit or behaviour pattern that is working well for you. If you have elements in your life that return, year after year, that are serving you well and are supporting you, then leave them alone. Trust the process. You don't need to start frantically tidying away parts of you which may no longer feel useful; perhaps they are providing a safe winter habitat for other parts of you. It's tempting to radically overhaul ourselves, strip everything away, be the neatest, trimmest, most severely pruned version of ourselves, especially in a society that demands change on the crest of a new year. What if we reject that? What if we leave our personal perennials alone and look forward to welcoming them back when they choose to emerge again? Perhaps we can accept the messy parts of ourselves and know that they are doing us good.

In contrast to perennials, we *are* encouraged to prune our roses in January/February. The advice is that modern roses can be cut back hard, whilst older varieties are more gently pruned. I love the metaphorical idea of removing thorny issues as we plan for our year ahead. Anything sharp that can spike us – self-criticism, self-doubt, fears and a lack of confidence – we can cut those right out of our plans for the year ahead and focus on looking forwards.

Meanwhile, the reminder that older roses need to be treated more gently resonates with my inner psychologist. We all have established thought patterns or behaviours that are acquired in our early years and then well-trodden into our psyche, and these require gentler handling. Just as we cannot grab a thicker, thornier branch because we are likely to prick ourselves, we need to handle these older, thornier issues with compassion. We can take extra care around our thickest thorns, testing what happens when we handle them with softness, gently snipping them away in order to allow for new growth and bigger blooms, in a way that is comfortable. We can deal with our thorniest issues, without hurting ourselves, and winter provides the space to do so.

We know that in order to bloom in spring, we need to rest, restore and plan, and this lesson comes directly from our gardens. In order to provide the fantastic floral displays of spring, many bulbs need to chill out. Literally. Flowers such as dahlias, daffodils and tulips will take what's known as a chill period for 12 to 14 weeks before beginning to flower. A hormone called abscisic acid (ABA) is released as the temperatures start to drop at the beginning of winter and then gradually loses potency across the season. As ABA, which inhibits leaf and stem growth, starts to leave a plant's system, it will push out new growth, which appears at the start of spring. In the same way, we can use a chill-out period at the start of winter to reflect and recover and then gently start to grow our ideas and plans as we move towards spring.

When plants are in their own personal chill-out period, the focus is not on what is above ground, but rather below. They use this period of dormancy to establish a root system that will support them for long-lasting blooms come spring. By paying attention to their foundations and building the strength of their roots, these plants are focusing on what will support them for the year ahead. Taking time to establish our own roots and to reflect, plan and plot aligns us with nature and allows us to create something long-term and sustainable. If we were to rush straight into *doing*, then we would produce something that could not last or thrive.

We have to consider the environment in which we are establishing our plans. Although the least 'showy' part of our gardens, it is the soil that takes centre-stage in winter, acting as a hive of activity. The soil breaks down organic matter, releasing enriching nutrients essential for plant growth and adding welcome richness to the soil. The advice in winter is to not turn the soil too often, in order to avoid losing heat, which is needed to continue to break down the organic matter and create rich and valuable compost. The same is true of us.

Throughout the rest of the year, we will gather some of our own organic matter. Life events, lessons learned, experiences had; the more positive and healing sitting alongside the harsher and tougher. All of these mix together and get broken down and processed, ready to be used as nourishment for the planting of our future dreams. This is why gentle sifting and only occasional turning is better for us. We don't get the best out of the compost of our year if we start sieving it too vigorously or endlessly raking over it. We don't have to solve or resolve everything in earliest winter, ready to start our new year with a clean slate. If we can sit with these lessons then we are better able to learn from them and use them for the future.

Winter may appear to be our garden's quietest season, but it's also a beautiful reminder of the cyclical nature of life. Beneath the frost, the plants, soil and wildlife are hard at work, ensuring a renewed burst of energy when the warmer days return. Embracing this season and its subtle rhythms fosters a deeper appreciation for the resilience and wonder of nature and of ourselves.

Mary Walton Upchurch, a landscape architect and author, claims that the best gardens are at their most beautiful in winter.[8] What makes a garden beautiful is the fundamental structure, which, although we can sense it in every season, becomes more prominent in winter. Without the distraction of fronds and foliage, we can see the shape and architecture of a garden, and it is the stripped-back season of winter that reveals the underneath. Everything from walls, hedges, walkways and steps can be seen more clearly and therefore appreciated. The same can be said of our trees and plants. When bared and exposed, these trees reveal their branches, barks and shapes. We become aware of interesting features on the trees themselves, without the distraction of the leaves and flowers that may initially take our attention in other seasons. There is strength in vulnerability, and whilst others may see these trees as lesser in winter, we should appreciate them for their simple elegance. It can be an uncomfortable truth that we can distract ourselves with the outside extras and neglect to appreciate the beauty of our foundations and structure. Winter asks us to consider: what is *our* fundamental structure showing us? What do we notice about ourselves when we are stripped of distractions and stand as we are? What happens when we reconnect with the very essence of ourselves? Can we appreciate our beauty in every season?

The work of nature photographers highlights the astonishing phenomenon of 'glowing' seedheads. When seedheads dry out, their translucent nature allows them to reflect sunlight from various angles, making them appear to sparkle or glow. Leaving the dry seedheads on plants, such as teasels, over winter allows their unusual aesthetic to be showcased, providing a warming aura on the chilliest of winter days. Which part of yourself can you let glow over winter? What reflects your sunshine from every angle? What allows you to showcase unexpected beauty? Learning to appreciate and trust our beauty in every season is not about aesthetics or what others define as beautiful. Beauty arises in unexpected places. Technically these seedheads, which provide such a glorious glow, could be considered spent. They have served their purpose and are now dried out. However, they offer seeds for future growth and so winter is inviting us to reflect on what we have learned from that which is now spent. What has the past given us which may boost or nourish our future? What gentle glow will light the next stage of our path?

It isn't fanciful to believe winter is asking us these questions; we are being offered invitations to reflect and reconsider at every turn. Whenever we spend even a few moments connected to nature in winter, we are inspired to reconnect with the ideas and values of our authentic selves. We are all glorious and beautiful; we can all gently glow.

Snow in a winter garden

I have a love-hate relationship with snow. Rumours of snow can cause a squirmy flurry of chionophobia (fear of snow) in my stomach and see me anxiously scanning weather forecasts. It is not the snow itself I don't like, but rather the feeling of being trapped. The UK is not fantastically equipped to deal with snow, meaning it doesn't take much for everything to grind to a halt. If I had to describe my ideal snow then it would be 'pretty but not inconvenient'. I can admire the niveous glow of startling white on the ground but I do prefer when it doesn't hang around. If the snow doesn't settle then I am delighted, my relief a sharp counterpoint to the disappointment on children's faces, holding their hands out to capture a snowflake which disappears on their palm, leaving only a speck of moisture as proof it was ever there.

That said, snow has its uses. I fell unexpectedly in love with snow when I lived in a rented two-bed Victorian house which was permanently freezing cold, no matter how high the thermostat and heating bill ran. One day, I swung my legs out of bed and realized I felt warm. In fact, my house was toasty for the first time. A thick blanket of snow had covered the roof and provided much-needed insulation overnight. This surprising gift of warmth, which continued for over a week as the snow continued to fall, was even more delightful for its unexpectedness, and I developed a newfound respect for the usefulness of snow.

Much as the snow protected me and my home, snow also holds a benefit for our gardens. Snow acts as an insulating blanket, protecting plants from extreme cold temperatures by trapping air within its flakes, which can be beneficial for most hardy plants. The sight of my garden after snow fills my heart with something exciting and childlike. I particularly enjoy the hush. The world is muffled by this covering and I love opening the window and hearing . . . nothing. My favourite is seeing snow in the moonlight. It is as though I get a sneak peak of something that the world won't see until the morning. Like peeling back a corner of wrapping paper, realizing what's underneath and waiting to see others' reactions.

Aristotle is quoted as saying, 'To appreciate the beauty of a snowflake, it is necessary to stand out in the cold.'[9] Although the origin of this statement is somewhat contested, whoever said it first, there is truth in it. I used to think snow was the type of weather perfectly described by the Icelandic term *gluggaveður*, which translates as 'window weather', i.e. weather that is best enjoyed through a window when one is cosy, warm and dry indoors. Snow used to be something I mainly observed anxiously through my weather app, but getting outside in the snow has taught me to appreciate it more. I like walking in snow; weirdly the weather often feels warmer after snow and I enjoy the freshness that it carries in the air.

I have also realized that there is no blanket term 'snow' but rather many different varieties. The Scottish word 'feefling' describes the flurry of light snow that often predicts a heavier snowfall is en route. Feefling snow is not like the movies. It isn't big, fat flakes falling and settling but rather it swirls, whisks and darts. Feefling snow is not at all calm and serene; the flakes move with a wild energy, as though they know that their very existence is about to cease and so they are trying to avoid falling to the earth. There's something so disorganized and chaotic about this lighter snow and it is mesmerizing to watch.

I have made my peace with snow. A little preparation prevents me feeling trapped or uncomfortable and I now see snow for the gift it is. There is a reminder that nature is more powerful than my plans. If I am supposed to speak at a conference or travel somewhere and it snows, then so be it. It's out of my control and there is something very liberating about letting go and trusting the process. Of course, it can be irritating and challenging when plans are disrupted, but I find that snow-acceptance has changed my attitude overall. I counter feeling trapped by getting out in the snow wherever I can. I gather supplies and stock the freezer. I go to the library and stockpile books. I send a video of our snow to my friend Bruce in Canada purely for comedy value, knowing that our few centimetres cannot compete with the several inches of snow that he will be facing.

I approach snow with a temperament more befitting the weather. I cover myself in a blanket of calm and hush, I face a bright white sheet where busy calendar plans used to sit and I embrace the snow as it falls. The snow in my garden often stays long after it has been driven into grey slush on the roads. It offers a small pocket of glittering calm once the world has resumed normality. I treasure that parcel of calm that sits outside my back door and continue my daily morning potter. The gifts of a winter garden unfold in all weathers and we can welcome them by being with them. Grab a cuppa and come join me outside. Let's treasure hunt together.

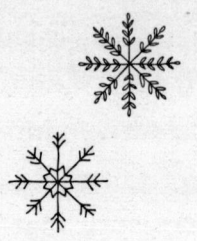

Chapter 15:
The practical preparations for winter

There is a process in farming called 'brooding'. A brooder is used to keep chicks warm in the coldest months during the most critical part of their development. Essentially it is a safe space for chicks to grow, learn and develop, with an infra-red heat lamp gently keeping them warm, ensuring the chicks and their surroundings are comfortable.

In researching this (easily my favourite piece of research because of the endless pictures of fluffy baby chicks), I discovered two core components in brooding. Firstly, as long as you check in regularly, the chicks will let you know exactly what they need and you can avoid any issues. For example, if the brooder heat source is too strong, then the chicks won't get close to it and you'll find them all huddled away from the heat. If the surrounding room or barn is too cold, then you will find it near impossible to shift the chicks from under the heat source. Secondly, you need to prepare your brooder early so that everything is in place for the moment the chicks hatch.

Without proper preparation, the chicks will experience a shock that leaves them uncomfortable, unhealthy and unable to cope. Checking in to see what we need and preparing for the season: two lessons that benefit us all.

When we are coming into winter, we need to prepare so that we can have the best season ahead. Whilst we cannot plan for every scenario, we can plan for the probable and for the very certain fact that winter is coming. Ignoring it, wishing it away and bemoaning it all require energy and become a drain on our resources. However, with a little preparation, a little setting up of our own brooder, we can absolutely grow, nurture and thrive our way through winter, discovering bursts of joy along the way.

Our preparations allow us to uncover our own version of winter magic. There is no definitive checklist, nor a tick-box exercise which on completion guarantees happiness. Our emotions, like the weather, are supposed to fluctuate in winter. However, preparation allows us to overcome the challenges and leads us to a new perspective: a lighter, more hopeful, more soulful way of seeing a different winter. A winter that steals our breath as we gaze at clear skies, frosted berries, heart-shaped leaves kissed with hoarfrost and murmurations worthy of an orchestral backing track. All of the gifts of winter lie at our feet. We need to prepare in order to open them.

The very act of planning and preparation engages several areas of the brain, including our prefrontal cortex. This is the executive decision-maker of the brain and is key in problem-solving and impulse control, which are particularly useful skills during the chaos of festive shopping and being in environments filled with temptation. There are wider brain benefits of planning too, including better memory, better mental health, lower stress and higher levels of neuroplasticity. By routinely planning and organizing, we enhance our brain's flexibility and efficiency. This also explains why reflection without direction can be so problematic; ruminating without any planning or organizing of our thoughts leaves us feeling jumbled and overwhelmed.

Whatever our brain practises and rehearses will build and strengthen neuro-connections, the brain's pathways of thought. Our brain is always looking to be the most efficient, so if there is a well-worn path then it will routinely choose that path. For example, if every time you hear the word 'winter' you think, 'Ugh, I hate winter,' your brain will automatically make that association and flood you with thought patterns and hormones to ensure that, yes, you really *do* hate winter. However, if you can plan and organize your neural pathways to look for the gifts of winter, then your brain is going to reward you with what you need to feel amazing, calm, secure and happy. This is why a little preparation goes a long way. This isn't about kidding yourself or denial; this is about rewiring your brain to have a happier and healthier winter.

A *genkan* is an entryway in a Japanese building where guests remove their shoes. When you enter a *genkan*, you will notice that all the shoes are lined up facing the door. This is a tiny act of preparation that allows guests to smoothly slide their feet into their shoes and be facing the right way when it is time to leave. Turning our shoes to face the door isn't an onerous or burdensome task, but it is a great example of how one small habitual act can remove a tiny bit of friction from our day, making the next part just that little bit easier. The same is true of preparing for winter. We don't need onerous or overly ambitious preparations, but small, simple shifts that remove friction and allow us to enjoy the season.

We can think of winter preparation just as a bird builds its nest. Birds won't try to build the whole structure in one day. Instead, a bird takes around three weeks to gather twigs, feathers and fur, collecting a little bit here and there, creating a 'cup' of grasses and twigs, then camouflaging it with moss and mud. Quite the comfy bed.

In order to avoid adding any unnecessary friction to a season that is encouraging us to move with ease, we too can prepare little and often. There are small steps we can take to make winter a little easier on us every year.

Our first act of preparation to remove friction is to prepare our mindset. We already touched on how we are primed by the media and marketing stunts, such as Blue Monday, to feel very negative towards winter. The semantics matter, and it is important that we pay attention to the words we use, not only when we describe winter to others, but when we think about the season ourselves. The words we use will activate certain parts of the brain and result in either positive or negative responses.[1] This is not about 'thinking positively' and never letting a negative word cross our minds, as our brains are equipped to handle and decipher variance and nuance. However, if there is an automatic response to winter that is habitual, rather than factual, then we need to address it. When we balance out our thoughts against winter with more neutral tones and allow ourselves to look for the positives, we make space to appreciate winter, and our brains will reward us for it.

I used to work in central London and, as a quiet country mouse, I wasn't immediately won over by the big city, which I found overwhelming, noisy and dirty. When I noticed these thoughts creeping in, I told myself that London was beautiful and set myself a challenge to see something beautiful every day. By setting that challenge, I deliberately walked through London seeing the good in the city. I noticed flowers wrapping themselves around the gates of giant office blocks. I noticed ornate carvings in stone works. I noticed that someone had put smiley-face stickers on every bus stop near my work. I noticed gorgeous, touching and loving messages on gravestones as I took a shortcut through a cemetery. I made myself look for the good and I relished my daily challenge of finding something beautiful every day (something I continue to this day, more than 10 years on).

> **Activity: Look for what's beautiful**
>
> Can you set yourself a challenge to see something beautiful in winter every day? Maybe keep notes on your phone or have a specific journal dedicated to capturing winter's striking beauty. We can find beauty in the everyday: the smile of a stranger, the sharing of an umbrella, the steam from a warming cup of coffee. Perhaps the spectacular sunrise you got up early to see, or the glossy chestnuts that you foraged for your table. Whatever it is, keep a note of all the beauty winter presents to you throughout the season and review your list whenever you need a mood boost.

A negative slant

Whilst writing this book, winter has been front and foremost in my mind and I've become hyper-aware of the attitudes and narratives about winter that surround us. It is not an exaggeration to say that we are bombarded by negative messaging from every angle. TV adverts, social media platforms, colleagues, even family, friends and neighbours. Nobody seems to offer anything positive and we are swimming in a sea of others' negativity. Emotions are contagious; we feel more negative when surrounded by others' negativity, and in a season when we are more reflective and thoughtful, it is important to channel the direction of our thinking more positively.

> **Activity: Balance the messaging**
>
> Can you seek out and connect with someone who enjoys the season? Who in your circle loves winter? What is their energy? Who do you know that radiates the warmth of the season? Perhaps you can start a conversation with those around you about the positives to balance some of the negatives? Perhaps that conversation can be included in your winter beauty journal.

Easing financial friction

We all have different incomes, different budgets, different constraints and different expenses so of course there is no 'one size fits all' when it comes to finances. However, one action that seems to benefit everyone is a little preparation.

Financial planning of any kind can feel a bit overwhelming. Money is extremely personal and I am not a financial advisor; I can only share here what works well for me, and that is looking ahead to winter. If you are reading this in the middle of winter, then use both your experiences from this winter and looking ahead to inform your choices.

My financial preparations start by working backwards. I consider what are the costs that would make winter cosier and easier for me, and then work my way back to any decisions and choices that I need to make *now* to support that. December is one of those months when everything seems due all at once. My professional accreditation renewals, my car tax, insurance and MOT, Christmas and all its associated costs, plus a lot of friend and family birthdays . . . it adds up to a very expensive month. Then there are the costs of winter itself. The increased energy bill plus any extras that I want for my retreat such as a new blanket, a snuggly jumper or a new candle for hygge days.

Whatever the costs are, I prepare for them as much as I can throughout the year so that there are no surprises. As ideas go, saving for items is not revelationary and it isn't always possible. But even a small saving can make a surprising difference to how we feel about winter. We can expect and therefore accept scarcity in winter but it doesn't need to be this way. There can be abundance and indulgence and lots of fun to be had, created by easing our financial strain as much as possible.

I put something aside every month which I don't touch until December. These days I do it all in an app, but when I started, I had a biscuit tin that I would put cash into every month. Saving even £5 per month meant I had £60 by the time December arrived, which made life just a little easier. I continue to save towards winter every month of the year. I wanted to change the narrative and mark the start of winter with a positive celebration, rather than with restriction and worry. A little planning helped me to do just that.

> 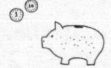 **Activity: Financial planning for winter**
>
> What expenses can you see ahead? What do you want to pay for that will enable you to have a more easeful winter? What can you gift yourself to mark the start of the season? Try to gather actual numbers and data so that you have exact figures to work with. Make a list of everything you would like to pay for over winter, then gradually tick it off throughout the year as you save the money. Seeing it written down makes it less intimidating and more tangible and gives a sense of achievement.

Winding down at work

For most of my career, I never really wound down for the holidays. I used to crash into Christmas at full pelt, coming to a screeching halt straight from the ward or office (job depending), and would experience the start of winter in a state of jangled nerves. Then one year I just . . . didn't. Where I could, I decided to deliberately wind down ahead of the new season starting. When people were requesting meetings that I had the calendar but not the cognitive capacity for, I replied saying, 'Can we reconvene when I have more headspace and can look at this with fresh eyes?' I don't think a single person pushed back or said no. In fact, many expressed relief at coming to it with a fresh mindset in a few weeks, rather than trying to make half-hearted progress at a time when they had little left in the tank.

Research published by the *Journal of Happiness Studies* found that it takes around eight days for us to let go of our responsibilities and stresses when we take a break.[2] This means that if we can start a gentle wind-down ahead of winter, then we can intentionally step into the season, ready to embrace the hush. Of course, for many of us, especially those working in retail or healthcare, winter may be a time when our workload drastically increases, and this makes it even more important to embrace the hush so we can deal with the rush. We can use that restorative invitation from winter to help us counter the increased pressure we are met with at work. We don't need time off work to start a winter wind-down, but we do need to pile less on our days. If our work demands increase, we can balance that by reducing external pressures. We can plan more winter retreat time, at the end of busy days. We can manage our inputs and ensure a post-work wind-down to balance and restore our energies.

When it comes to work, we need to be realistic about how much energy we have and what we want to take into the new year. It's better for us, better for our colleagues and better for our work.

> **Activity: Reducing the demand**
>
> What is one small adjustment you can make to your work or other daily demands that would serve you well in winter?
>
> Is there one demand that you could let go of or reduce temporarily to allow you to balance the other pulls on your time and attention?
>
> Are you making any unreasonable demands of yourself that you can replace with compassion and understanding instead? Can you reach the same goals with gentle kindness as your guide?

Taking care of your health

Taking care of your physical health is one of the best ways to boost your winter wellbeing. We tend to discuss our mental health and our physical health as though they are two separate entities, whereas the reality is that they are intertwined and we cannot separate them. We already know the benefits of making adjustments in order to keep movement in our winter routines, but there are other aspects to consider.

Winter is often a time of year when we are surrounded by food that we wouldn't typically eat, in quantities that we would normally baulk at. It can feel impossible to escape as colleagues, supermarkets and family members push large tins of chocolates, boxes of mince pies and bottles of alcohol our way. We can feel as though saying no to such proffered goodies is showing a lack of holiday spirit and as though we are somehow spoiling things for others, but it is us that returns home demotivated, listless and depressed.

We don't address this much in society but alcohol *is* a depressant. It literally depresses your parasympathetic nervous system, which means you are squashing down the part of your brain that is going to keep you happy, relaxed, able to think clearly and problem-solve. Given the propensity for many of us to struggle with winter blues or the more pervasive SAD, it makes sense to limit alcohol over winter. A lot of social occasions can prompt heavier drinking than we are used to and we see people use these as an excuse to drink more often and at unusual times of the day. However, by being mindful of our intake, we are protecting our own mental health and therefore our winter wellbeing.

Nowadays, there are so many fantastic low-alcohol alternatives and 'fake' drinks, which means that even if everyone else is having a G&T and you'd prefer not to, you can still join in, only with an alcohol-free version. If you are thinking, 'Gosh, this sounds absolutely miserable,' then don't be mistaken, I'm not saying you should never drink over winter, but it is good to consider limiting alcohol as part of your winter preparation. If you dampen all your support mechanisms, then you will dampen your mood, which won't serve you well. Your brain is in a space where it wants to reflect, consider, plan and ponder. If you drink your brain into a depressed state, then all this natural reflection is going to be through a more negative and pessimistic filter.

Speaking of drinking, winter is also a time to pay attention to hydration. Dehydration sets in when the body loses more water than it takes in; however, it's easy to lose track, especially when the temperatures drop. As we sweat less in winter, we can forget to hydrate or believe that our thirst is adequately quenched. Putting the heating on can cause a drier environment, which can lead to increased water loss simply from breathing.[3] Even minor dehydration, the level at which we begin to feel thirsty, can cause challenges to memory and concentration and lead to lower mood. Drinking water throughout the day is a very effective way to improve your health and wellbeing over winter. If a cool glass of water doesn't hold much appeal, then hot drinks such as herbal teas or hot water with lemon or ginger can be a good alternative, keeping us hydrated *and* warm.

All of these practical preparations are small but impactful actions we can take as we move into winter. If we can see these as part of the ritual of entering the season, the setting up of our brooder, then we are preparing both our body and our mind to experience the greatest sense of winter wellbeing that we can. Much like turning our shoes to face the door, these small steps will remove some of the friction and allow us to move through the season with ease.

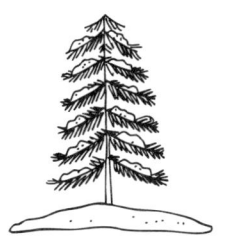

Chapter 16:
A beginning, a middle and an end

As with every season, there is a distinct beginning, middle and end to winter. The beginning is the planning phase, the middle is the being phase and the end is the preparing phase. In the planning phase, we pause, reflect and think. We journal and create and sketch out our year ahead, without launching into anything. It is a gentle easing into the season and it is my favourite part. It offers a reprieve from the rush and the chaos. It is when we are gifted time to think and reflect, without needing to *do*.

Remember in our reworking of the year (see pages 11–14), the starting gun doesn't go off until April, so we have three leisurely months before we need to start the *doing*. This first phase is the perfect time to plan.

Planning for the in-between days

We can be so busy planning our festivities that we forget about the in-between, which is offered to us in the first week of winter following the solstice. The in-between is the time that sits between Christmas and New Year. When I was little, these days were characterized by grown-ups asking each other what day it was, overeating chocolates out of tins and half-watching truly awful movies on TV. But what I remember most is the feeling of waiting around. These weren't productive days, they felt wasted, but not deliciously so. There can be something truly indulgent in choosing to waste time every now and then; it can be a wonderful treat. However, the opposite is true of time being wasted unintentionally. Those days where we want to do something but don't seem able to settle to anything, see us feeling markedly dissatisfied at the end of the day.

The in-between can be a real gift if we plan for it. It can provide a space to lay the foundations of a good winter early on in the season. It can be a time for reflection, for daydreaming, for reading, for doodling. It can be a time for gentle, cosy get-togethers. It can be a time to tune in daily. How you set yourself up for this, how you reconnect to what works for you and those closest to you, can set the tone for the planning phase of your winter.

Disturbing the peace

As we settle into the hush and prepare to sink into a season of restoration and reflection, we are presented with New Year's Eve. I must confess, I am not a big New Year's Eve person in the traditional sense. Not because I don't like celebrating, but because the New Year's Eve celebrations that we are told we 'should' have are just not my bag.

I have experienced some fabulous, fun and frivolous New Year's Eve celebrations, but I have also held back a friend's hair as she hurled into some poor person's front garden, pleaded with taxi after taxi as they refused to take us home and shivered in outfits only suitable for the overpriced and overstuffed venue we have just left, definitely not for early-hour temperatures of 1 January.

For me, the biggest consideration for New Year's Eve is about how I want to start the new year. The idea of going to bed very late, waking early (I've never mastered a lie-in, plus I have dogs) and feeling foggy-headed, bleary and knackered all day makes me feel sad and thwarted. Getting home in the early hours and starting the year cold, tired and grumpy is not how I want to feel in that first phase of winter.

The older I get, the less time and patience I have for wasting energy in ways I don't want to. I am all for making an effort with friends and connecting, but as someone who doesn't want to have a drunken night out, I have realized that there are so many different ways to engage in New Year's Eve celebrations that don't make you 'boring'. I used to think there was something wrong with me or that I was a massive killjoy, but the more I tuned into winter's energy, the more I saw why these noisy, drunken celebrations were not for me. They clash with the energy of winter itself.

I started to realign the energy of my New Year's Eve about 10 years ago. I went to see my parents early in the evening and sensed that they did not want to stay up until midnight and were waiting because they felt they had to celebrate. I said to my dad, 'I think you're being super-polite, but why don't we celebrate together now? What are we waiting for?' I don't think it was even 8.30pm before we were toasting the new year, sharing our hopes and intentions for the coming year and reflecting on what we were thankful for from the year just gone. It was a wonderful and very happy evening and I joined in the toast with sparkling elderflower in a champagne glass. I felt part of it, but I didn't have to drink (I, along with every neuroscientist I know, avoid alcohol). We hugged, we smiled, we laughed and I left them to it at about 10pm. I could see they were delighted to have celebrated and shared some good times, but I also saw the lights click off before I had even reversed my car off their drive. They were happy, I was happy. Now to start my new year.

I drove home and let myself into the quiet. I lit candles, changed into my softest and comfiest outfit and completed a gentle yoga practice. I had the television on, showing the festivities but without the sound, and had beautiful soft music playing, uplifting and calming my heart and soul. My yoga practice ended as the clock struck midnight (not planned but immensely satisfying) and I sat on my mat, watching the fireworks, feeling unbelievably relaxed, serene, grounded and content. I then went to bed and slept for a solid eight hours, an unheard-of pleasure for me. I awoke the next day feeling the most amazing I had felt for months and it was a fantastic energy with which to start the new year.

When I recount that story to others, not a single person tells me that I missed out. Instead, they make a wistful noise and say, 'Oh, that sounds perfect,' and tell me that they are going to do something similar for their next New Year celebrations. You see, many of us don't want to follow the 'traditional' path of drinking until we're ill and starting the new year feeling atrocious. We want something different and it's all available to us. We can carry whatever energy we want from one year to the next.

Other times, I have celebrated by driving to a beach for sunrise, watching the first daybreak of the year whilst huddled under a blanket. I have stayed with friends and giggled like teenagers at a sleepover. I have taken part in kitchen discos and danced until dawn, spending the next day sleepy but happy and contented from the connection with those I love. Like Christmas, we can tune in year on year and see what we want to create for ourselves. We don't need to subscribe to one idea of New Year.

> **Activity: How will you begin the year?**
>
> Take some time to think about your New Year's Eve and how you want to begin the year. It is never too late to celebrate the start of the year and welcome that energy, whether you do that on the first day of the year or at any point during winter. You create your celebrations and can plan them exactly as you want to. What will your celebration look like this year?

A different resolution

Although we are told it is just another day, I do like the symbolism of a new year. That feeling of a clean slate. I love a goal, a plan, an intention, seeing a blank page in a notebook and the endless possibilities that it holds. For me, the start of a new year is the ultimate blank page and I am excited to get scribbling.

Over the last few years, there seems to have been a real trend of dismissing New Year's resolutions. Whereas magazines used to be full of articles telling you 'how to make next year YOUR year' and encouraging you to 'smash your goals', the rhetoric these days seems to be the antidote. Instead of posts pushing you to change, there seems to be a lot more focus on being OK exactly as you are, self-acceptance and focusing on the positives you already have in your life, as opposed to striving for more. Seeing the rhetoric shift has been like watching a pendulum swing from one extreme to the other. Whilst I think this recent narrative *can* be a very positive message, I also think it can be demotivating and misleading. Our brains like a goal, a plan, a pathway. Without one, they will wander off on their own and make wayward decisions. You are going to fall into habits, patterns and behaviours regardless, so you may as well take control of them. However, this process doesn't need to be self-critical or aggressive. You can be intensely grateful for what you have, whilst also seeking more of what will make you happy and fulfilled. This is why the planning phase of winter is so important. We can connect to our core values and consider what truly matters to us and how to get more of it into our year in a way that is manageable and restorative, rather than challenging and draining.

Social media highlights the resharing of memes saying things like, 'Flowers don't bloom in winter; you shouldn't expect to either' and the implication of these is that it's OK to slow down and catch your breath, and that is so true. But we know there is a big difference between blooming and growing. Maybe winter isn't the time to emerge with a loud blousy 'TA DA!' of a bloom. We know from nature that these won't last in winter, as the weather conditions cannot sustain them. But these blooms do start growing and developing throughout winter. We can learn so much from this cycle of nature. It doesn't make sense to loudly shout in a season of quiet reflection, which is why highly demanding New Year's resolutions can feel so jarring. They are misplaced. But there is room for a different resolution, one of continual growth.

Resolutions have gained a bad reputation over the years, as people used them as an opportunity for self-criticism and judgement, whilst striving towards unrealistic targets and ideas. It always strikes me as odd that so many people who drink and stay up late on New Year's Eve set a New Year's resolution to go running, starting on 1 January. Literally every aspect of that behaviour is setting them up to fail. They'll be tired, dehydrated, lacking in energy and cold and their parasympathetic nervous system will be depressed, meaning they'll feel aches and pains more acutely. Essentially, the worst conditions in which to go for a run. New Year's resolutions don't need to be completed on 1 January, nor should we aim to start everything all at once.

We can use winter's planning phase to build not only our resolutions, but what we need to make them work. James Clear, author of *Atomic Habits*, states that we don't rise to the level of our goals, but fall to the level of our systems.[1] So many resolutions are made without systems in place to support them. Continued failure, year in, year out, is not appealing and so eventually we give up on New Year's resolutions, declaring them a waste of time. However, wandering aimlessly into the year, feeling stuck by old habits and unable to instigate new goals is also not a healthy way to start the year. When we think of our resolutions, we need to see the winter months as the time for sowing seeds; building the systems to support our goals.

Making it happen

One of my favourite pieces of advice about waiting for the right time is: don't. Make it work in the wrong time, then experience how easy it is when the time is right. You will already have the systems in place to support you and everything will feel infinitely easier. Let's say you want to write a novel but you have many other pulls on your time and energy (full-time work, raising children, other responsibilities, taking care of an elderly parent, etc.). If you can make time for writing three times per week despite all that, even if it's only to write one sentence, one thought or one paragraph, then think how easy that three times per week will feel when you are less overwhelmed. You already have a three-times-per-week system in place, so when the circumstances change, that system and the progress you achieve within it will get easier.

The same is true of New Year's resolutions. January is not the best time to try to make big dramatic shifts, either from an energy- or cognitive-capacity perspective. However, it is the perfect time to gently start laying systems in place and reaping the rewards of those throughout the year.

Activity: Setting up your systems

What would you like to achieve this year? Be sure that your goals for the year are centred around you. Anything that is not focused on you is a task not a goal. If you immediately thought, 'I want to replace the garage roof,' then that is a great task to achieve, but it isn't a goal about *you*. What do *you* want to achieve? What would make your life easier? What would make your soul dance? What do you want future you to feel happy about?

Once you have a goal that focuses on you, think about the system you need to set up to achieve it. What do you need to put in place, arrange or make space for that would allow you to achieve your goal? Also consider what the bare minimum is to achieve that goal. For example, I want a regular yoga practice and so I have a daily goal to sit on my yoga mat and take five deep breaths. Sometimes this leads to further practice, but sometimes all I have time to do is deliberately sit and take five breaths and that's enough for me. My goal isn't to have the most difficult or social-media-worthy practice, but to have consistency. Five breaths every day meets that goal. It's a bare-minimum system that sets me up for success.

Take a moment to write down your goal and your bare-minimum system to support it. With your planning done, you are now ready for the middle phase: being.

The being phase

The being phase is probably the most challenging in winter. As we begin to restore our energy and make plans, our doing selves want to get going. We itch to get started on projects and move things along, and we really have to hold back from 'doing' and instead sit in 'being'. We often realize that our motivation and energy are not quite aligned, and the middle phase of winter offers us a space to rebalance the two. We can be with our plans, ruminate on them, develop them, mature them. This part of the season is our time to recharge and feel that gentle and restorative seasonal energy thrum through us, replenishing us with what we need, before moving into the higher-energy months. Starting to *do* too soon is a mistake and one I have fallen foul of.

I have definitely had ideas, got excited about my plans and started to *do*, only to run out of steam and not finish them, leaving me disappointed and disheartened. Staying in the middle phase for longer allows me to fully recharge so that I have the energy and stamina for the year ahead and whatever I hope to achieve. This being phase is the equivalent of having a nourishing meal over grabbing a snack bar. The full meal is the one which will sustain us, replenish us and revitalize us, whereas the snack bar gives us a small burst of energy that quickly fizzles out.

The being phase isn't sitting still, but rather gathering resources. If you are someone who typically runs at life, impatient for the next part, always rushing forwards, then the being phase of mid-winter is there just for you. It is a space to slow down and simply breathe. It is a space of no pressure. There are, of course, external pressures and deadlines throughout winter, but the being phase allows us to monitor our energy and achieve whilst prioritizing rest and realignment.

I often tell myself 'Not yet' in this phase. The doing will come, all too quickly. This phase is for developing the deepest connection to ourselves. We have set out our plans and our goals and now we wait. We simply be.

It doesn't come naturally to me but every time I make myself stop and be in this phase, I benefit. My mood is good, my year gets off to a better start. Inevitably, I discover a perfect time to begin a project, task or goal that definitely wasn't in the being phase. It's an incredibly powerful part of winter and I cherish it more for its challenge.

 Activity: Simply be with winter

What is an activity or goal that you are excited about, that you can sit with in the being phase? What can you do to be still with mid-winter and benefit from the recharging energy that this phase offers? What can you do to stop yourself rushing ahead? How can you ground yourself in simply being?

The final phase: preparing

The final phase of winter sees us preparing to leave the season, and it's the one I struggle with the most. As someone who used to wish away the season, it feels so strange that now it never feels long enough. I never thought I'd be reluctant to let go of winter, but I find it such a restorative season and I want to hold on to the peace, the warmth and the cosy pace that I develop across the three months for far longer. But, of course, it comes to a close.

They say everything happens for a reason and for a season. We are supposed to move through different phases. We are always evolving with different habits, different mindsets, a different sense of purpose. I can feel a bit adrift outside of winter but we must remember that we never stand alone, but with nature; and nature never stands still. Each blade of grass is growing and millions of creatures are moving, adapting and adjusting their routines to align with the seasons, and we must too. We must prepare to leave winter.

As winter ends, I experience feelings of gratitude mixed with sadness. I want to stay for ever in this gorgeous season that allows me to dream and plan, whilst prioritizing my health and wellbeing. Having wrapped my arms tightly around winter at the beginning, now that we reach the final preparing phase, winter delicately disentangles itself from my grip, giving me gentle nudges towards spring. Winter offers beautiful gifts, almost bribes, to move forwards. *See the cherry blossom?* winter asks. *That will only get more magnificent. Those gorgeous buds starting to open up will grow and develop their character once I move aside for spring.* This phase is a gentle warming-up. We can begin to do more, and the energy shifts beneath us, giving us more daylight from an earlier hour. The birds around us reacquaint themselves with their vocal cords and begin serenading us with an earlier dawn chorus. Winter's work is done and it hands the reins to spring. The preparing phase sees us begin to utilize that gentle wake-up, that shift, that slow ramp up towards the higher-energy frequency of spring.

My explorations of winter have led to the development of deep feelings and warm attachment to the season, but we don't have to let go of winter completely. It offers us learnings that we can all carry with us into other seasons; these are its parting gifts. It teaches us to approach each season without expectation. To look for the beauty of whatever season we are in, to pay attention to nature and to tune in to our energy. To not feel as though we have to be a certain way.

We can be present in the season around us as it is, not how we think it should be, or how we see it in our mind's eye. We can approach each day afresh. We can plug into the boundless energy of nature, knowing that it can offer all the hope, advice, space, lightness and grounding that we could ever need.

A letter to my future self

Every winter, I write a letter to myself which I won't open until 1 December, ready to begin my seasonal preparations. Although I author that letter, I typically completely forget what it contains and I look forward to seeing what advice my past self had for my current self. In my letter, I include a reflection on winter so far, what has worked and what hasn't, and I offer myself words of gentle encouragement. These words feel powerful, as they remain the same, regardless of how the year has gone. My letter provides me with a wonderful reminder to connect with activities, people and dreams that make me feel good, and it carries me into winter with optimism and warmth in my soul.

These letters serve a greater purpose; writing them provides a roadmap for the year ahead. Knowing where we want to go and what we want to achieve is helpful for our brains. Once we provide a direction of travel, then our brains will map the route accordingly. Without such a map, our brains will keep moving us forward but possibly not in the direction we want to go, and we may miss turnings and opportunities that were signposted for us. These letters serve as a manifestation of the year ahead. Manifestation can be wrongfully scorned as wishful thinking but the neuroscience supports it. Whilst simply wishing for something won't result in it happening, being able to envision your path and what you want your future self to be accomplishing primes your brain to look out for the relevant opportunities in the year ahead.

There are many tools and tips you can use to remind yourself of your journey and your hopes, but I recommend writing a letter to yourself and then leaving it until 1 December, just before winter arrives, so that you can guide yourself through winter and the year ahead. Fill that letter with love and compassion and engage in positive self-talk and encouragement for a future that is brimming with possibility. Your letter is not a place for threat or recrimination. There is no space for, 'You'd better have done this or else!' on your page. Instead, it is an embrace from past you, a nudge into the future, a reminder of what has worked well and what you might want to try again.

> **Activity: Write a letter to your future self**
>
> This is a letter that you will open on 1 December, or perhaps on the winter solstice if you prefer. A letter just for you and no one else.
>
> Appreciating that you may be reading this book after winter solstice or that you may not have the time or resources just now to write a letter, I have also written a letter to you. I hope that my words help you to prepare for your year, whether you are about to enter winter, a new year or a new phase. Whatever is ahead, these words are for you.

Dear Friend,

I hope this letter finds you well and that you are ready to embrace winter's hug, if you haven't already. Start by stopping. Take a breath, take a moment and tune in. What do you need right now? What is your body asking for? How is your energy at the moment? You may have had a wonderful year and be smiling broadly as you reflect, or you may be crawling to the finish line ready to put the year behind you. In all likelihood, you will have experienced a bit of both, some good and some bad. Be sure to bring both to mind; don't let the shadows of the darker times block out the rays of sunshine.

Whatever your year has brought you to date, know that winter is here for you, arms wide open, ready to embrace you and realign you with the heartbeat of nature. As you cross the threshold of winter, get ready to get cosy. The fire is lit, the fairy lights are twinkling, the kettle is on. If you're not getting 10,000 things done today, that is OK. Winter is a season of slowing down and hush. What noise can you let go of? What can you banish? What can you leave behind in the previous seasons that will allow you to sink into winter's embrace and recharge? What is not welcome in your winter this year?

You are not alone this season; winter is right here with you. Along every step of your journey, you will find winter a strong and supportive companion. Relax into winter's arms. Sink back. Close your eyes. Winter will hold you, heal you and restore you. You will grow and learn and plan, and before you know it, you will be stepping into spring re-energized and feeling renewed. Let winter take care of you now. You don't need to do anything other than become quiet and still enough to hear winter's whispers.

I do not know what your year ahead holds, but you do. Imagine yourself one year from now: happy, fulfilled and satisfied. What are you proud of doing or not doing? What have you carried and what have you released? What was one brave act that rewarded you for your courage?

You don't need to leap into action right now; this is not a call to arms. Rather, this is your period of reflection and planning, a time for ideas to bud and grow as you slowly unfurl and stretch towards the sunlight. This is your time; a time not to do but to think. What does the year ahead hold for you?

Whatever has happened this past year and whatever is next for you, take a moment to feel proud of yourself. Place your palm on your chest and feel the heartbeat that has carried you through this year. Whatever you are going through, thinking through or pushing through, know that we are in it together; my heart beats with yours.

Take excellent care of yourself, you are so worth it. Enjoy the might and momentum of winter; its strength is right behind you.

Thank you for reading my letter and my book. I sincerely hope you have a wonderful winter, set up with the tools and vision to carefully unwrap and treasure the gifts winter has just for you.

Take care, my friend, see you next winter.

Steph xxx

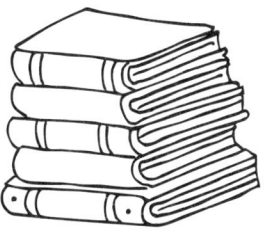

Epilogue:
The words of winter

A simple search for 'winter adjectives' presents us with a fairly miserable list: cold, bleak, dark, gloomy, dreary, sad, depressing and so on. Just reading these words can cause our mood and heart to sink. But the winter you and I see does not exist in these words. Where are the words for the winter full of magic, glitter, light, joy, connection and celebration? We need a new language for winter that allows us to describe the gifts of the season. As we change how we approach winter, the vocabulary we use needs to change with us.

We don't need to deny aspects of winter. As in any season, there are days where the words 'gloomy' and 'dark' are perfectly apt. But there are so many more days when the gifts of winter are unwrapped for us, and we need the language to share these with others.

The following offers some beautiful words to broaden our description of winter.

Yutori

The whole season of winter can be neatly summarized by the Japanese word *yutori* (ゆとり – pronounced 'yoo toh ree'). *Yutori* translates as 'space' or 'room to breathe'. It describes an intentional slowing down, a time without rushing, a time to be, to savour and appreciate the nature around us. *Yutori* encapsulates the very spirit of winter. It is not a time of stopping but a time of deliberate slowing. Taking this time to reconnect with and savour the nature around us allows us to realign with the season. It presents us with an amazing opportunity to explore the softness of a season that is often presented as harsh. If we can consider winter as our space in the year simply to be and to breathe, then it is our season of *yutori*.

Prinkling

Prinkling is a beautiful word to say, and it exactly fits the feeling it describes. Prinkling is the tingling sensation we get in our hands and feet as they begin to warm up after being out in the cold. The feeling of prinkling as we enter our homes after a winter walk is glorious, only enhanced by wrapping our hands around a mug of hot chocolate and revelling in the warmth of being indoors. That gentle thawing also describes the energy of winter. A season of slowly awakening, of warming and coming back to life. A re-energizing and recharging. It is not just our hands that prinkle; we can feel a sense of prinkling deep within our hearts and minds. Our plans, hopes and ambitions can prinkle throughout the season as we slowly warm up and prepare for the year ahead.

Lagom

The Swedish word *lagom* describes when something feels just right; neither too much nor too little. It fits perfectly in winter, particularly as part of our winter retreat havens, also known as 'hibernacles'. Hibernacle comes from the Latin word *hibernus*,[1] meaning wintery, and is the cosy space we create in our homes to be with winter and take a purposeful rest. When you have the set-up just right, your blanket is covering you, your tea is the perfect temperature, your book or favourite show has your attention, you have no stresses or worries and you are relaxed in the moment, know that winter is gifting you a moment of *lagom* within your very own hibernacle.

Ohana

When we think of winter, we may not immediately think of Hawaii, but the Hawaiian word *ohana* describes those closest to us, those friends who are like family. We have many English words, such as 'chosen family' or 'kin', but *ohana* represents a community comprised of those we care for and share with. It is our *ohana* that our brains want to connect with in winter. Traditionally a time for close clan gatherings, for story-telling around the fire, for sharing tales of the year just gone and planning together for the year ahead. There is no pressure in these groups; we can authentically be who we are, and our *ohana* understand and support us. Summer allows us to dance to bands with strangers in fields, and we can butterfly across our connections. In winter we want to sit with our *ohana*. Winter is the perfect time to gather those closest to you and enjoy the feeling of connection with people you can be yourself with.

Gemütlichkeit

The German word *gemütlichkeit* translates as cosiness and is defined by a feeling of warmth, cheer and a sense of belonging. We can feel *gemütlichkeit* when we spend time with others and feel connected with a community. The social acceptance and being safe and cosy together gives us a glorious feeling of wellbeing. There is a friendliness innate in *gemütlichkeit*, and we can snuggle into that contented cosiness together. This can also be paired with the Dutch word *gezelligheid*, which refers to a sense of shared closeness, contentment and conviviality. There is also an element of fun in *gezelligheid*. It can be a noisy night in the pub with friends, a natter around the kitchen table sharing stories and jokes or even laughing at a film together on the sofa. It doesn't need to be flash, but the sense of connection and fun builds on the social cosiness of *gemütlichkeit*, and we can feel confident and safe with our community of friends and family.

Trygghet

Speaking of safety, *trygghet* is another favourite winter word from Sweden and relates to a sense of safety and security. That feeling we get when we walk in the door after being outside, particularly in more challenging weather, and we get to close the door behind us and softly exhale. As we stand still and feel the welcoming embrace of our own space, we feel a sense of security and safety in being home, which is hard to describe in English. It's a feeling of certainty and trust. There is something beautiful about the sense of *trygghet* that winter can inspire in us.

Fàng xīn

The Mandarin Chinese words *fàng xīn* (pronounced 'fang shin') beautifully describe winter's invitation to relax and be at ease. They describe a sense of reassurance that stepping into winter offers us. There is a sense of trust inherent in *fàng xīn*, and winter provides us with that reassurance. As we ease into the hush, align with nature and trust the season, we can feel an affinity with winter that offers us what we need to recover from previous seasons. *Fàng xīn* is the feeling you get when you step into your winter retreat space, when you are not preoccupied, when you can relax and unwind your busy mind.

Confelicity

Confelicity is a beautiful word for winter as it describes the joy we can feel at seeing someone else's happiness. We may experience confelicity when we watch someone open a carefully selected present or see them relax and unwind during a hygge moment. I feel confelicity every time I see my dogs' paw prints in snow as they run around with renewed zest. I feel confelicity when I watch children walk past our window on the way to school, resembling puffed-up clouds in their coats, excitedly chattering with faces turned towards the sky to see the snow falling. Deliberately finding joy and happiness in another's joy or success is a beautiful feeling to cultivate. The world we live in encourages envy and competition with others. To feel joy because of someone else's success and happiness is a rebellion against this and leaves us feeling so much healthier and happier. Also, experiencing joy and happiness for others opens us up to many more ways to feel happy than just our own lives; there is a whole world out there that we can celebrate. Look for reasons to be happy for someone and you will experience a season, maybe even a lifetime, of confelicity which is good for you and good for others.

Peiskos

Peiskos[2] is a deeply satisfying Norwegian word to describe a deeply satisfying feeling. *Peiskos* is the contented, cosy feeling we get when sitting indoors enjoying the warmth of a fireplace. Fire holds a special place in winter. The use of fireplaces, chimeneas and candles means that winter is a season of flames, and the soft golden light of a fireplace matches the warmth it exudes. To come in from the cold and walk into a pub or café to see a welcoming warming fire, preferably with some sofas to flump onto, allows us to embrace *peiskos* at its best.

Self

Winter is the season of the self. Self-love, self-compassion, self-connection. It is not a selfish season but a season where we have permission to focus on ourselves. A season to be authentic. We have the hush, the headspace and the reflective mindset to explore ourselves and reconnect to our truest self. The definition of 'self' is a person's essential being that distinguishes them from others. We can get so caught up in the busyness of life that winter can provide a very welcome and necessary season of self. We don't have to withdraw from or forget others, but we can reconnect with and remember ourselves. If you have been focused on others within your family, your social circle or even online via social media, then winter is your time. Embrace your 'self' and pay renewed attention to who you are.

Acknowledgements

A massive thank you to my wonderful agent Kate Barker. Meeting Kate was a perfect example of serendipity in action and this book would not be in your hands without her. I want to also thank my incredible publishers, especially Ione, who was able to reach into my brain and see what I wanted to offer in this book, and her amazing team who made it happen, including Sukhmani, Katya, Nina, Ellie and Alice. I want to thank Victoria Roddam, who has been with me since the beginning and has been the number one cheerleader for my writing. Thank you for sticking with me, Victoria, even when I had no clue what I was doing and was probably *that* author. I am bolder and braver because of you.

I want to thank those of you who are holding this book. Special thanks to those who have ever muttered 'I hate winter,' yet still opened the pages and opened your hearts. I hope it serves you well and I hope it continues to help you fall in love with and benefit from winter. I hope you can enjoy and not endure this magical season.

I want to thank my gorgeous book club for being the most supportive group (even if we never actually discuss books!) and for cheering for me along the way. I want to thank my best friend, Emma, for supporting me not just with this book, but for my whole life since primary school. Also huge thanks to Odelia, for always being happy for me and for being a fellow lover of all things winter. I want to thank Bruce for sharing his harsh Canadian winters with me, but also for being the most fantastic friend and for listening to me talk about this book for years now (our friendship is the best holiday souvenir I have ever kept!). Of course, love and thanks also go to my mum and dad, Ros and Joe, for their ongoing support and encouragement.

I want to thank my girls for being my loyal furry office companions, being the best company and providing an endless supply of oxytocin. I want to thank Matt Clark, although thanks doesn't seem enough. Your support and love through everything *is* everything to me. Thank you Mr, you are simply amazing.

Lastly, I want to thank winter. Thank you for sticking with me, for forgiving me for being so rude about you when I struggled, thank you for showing me everything you had to offer and thank you for offering me the warmest hug through the coldest days. I will forever hold you in my heart.

Thank you. xxx

Endnotes

Introduction

1 Clare, H., *The Light in the Dark: A Winter Journal* (Elliott & Thompson Ltd, 2018).

Chapter 1: Making space for winter

1 Ipsos UK, 'Days may be getting shorter, but summer is still Britain's favourite season', www.ipsos.com (2024) [accessed 25 April 2025].

2 Austen, J., 'Letter to Cassandra (18 September 1796)', *Jane Austen Selected Letters 1796–1817*, ed. R. W. Chapman (The World's Classics, 1955), p. 9.

3 Met Office, 'When does spring start?', www.metoffice.gov.uk (2025) [accessed 25 April 2025].

4 Wikipedia, 'Fiscal year', www.wikipedia.com [accessed 25 April 2025].

Chapter 2: A winter mood

1. NHS Digital, 'Adult Psychiatric Morbidity Survey: Survey of mental health and welbeing, England, 2014', www.digital.nhs.uk (29 September 2016) [accessed 25 April 2025].

2. NutraIngredients Europe, 'Nearly half of UK adults unaware of gov's winter vit D guidelines, BNF survey finds', www.nutraingredients.com (2021) [accessed 25 April 2025].

3. Office for Health Improvement and Disparities, 'National Diet and Nutrition Survey', www.gov.uk (2016) [accessed 25 April 2025].

4. US National Institutes of Health, 'Vitamin D fact sheet for consumers', www.ods.od.nih.gov (2022) [accessed 25 April 2025].

5. NutraIngredients Europe, 'Nearly half of UK adults unaware of gov's winter vit D guidelines'.

6. Nuffield Health, 'Seasonal Affective Disorder: The Signs, symptoms, and treatments', www.nuffieldhealth.com (2023) [accessed 25 April 2025].

7. American Psychiatric Association, 'Seasonal Affective Disorder', www.psychiatry.org (2023) [accessed 25 April 2025].

8. US National Institutes of Health, 'Beat the winter blues', www.newsinhealth.nih.gov (2013) [accessed 25 April 2025].

Chapter 3: A shift in mindset

1. Peat, J., 'Man who coined the term "Blue Monday" apologises for making January more depressing', *Independent* (5 January 2018).

Chapter 4: Embracing a winter break

1. 'Summer Holiday', written by Bruce Welch and Brian Bennett.
2. Tripadvisor, 'Summer Travel Index 2023', www.tripadvisor.mediaroom.com (10 May 2023).
3. HSBC UK, 'Brits ditch the summer staycation for budget winter holidays abroad', www.abouthsbc.co.uk (2023) [accessed 25 April 2025].
4. Redbooth, 'Everybody's working for the weekend, but when do you actually get work done?', www.redbooth.com (15 November 2017).
5. Winter, M., 'Over 57 million days of annual leave went unclaimed in 2020 due to pandemic, study finds', *Daily Express* (28 July 2021).
6. Dykins, R., 'Half of working UK adults fail to take full annual leave allocation', www.globetrender.com (19 January 2023) [accessed 25 April 2025].

Chapter 5: A winter retreat at home

1. 'Hygge, n. & adj.', *Oxford English Dictionary*, www.oed.com [accessed 25 April 2025].

2   *Ibid.*

3   Visit Denmark, 'What is hygge?', www.visitdenmark.com [accessed 25 April 2025].

Chapter 6: A winter bedtime

1   Basile, L. M., 'Do we lose sleep to Seasonal Affective Disorder?', www.sleepfoundation.org (2022) [accessed 25 April 2025].

2   Seidler, A., *et al.*, 'Seasonality of human sleep: Polysomnographic data of a neuropsychiatric sleep clinic', *Frontiers in Neuroscience*, 17 (2023).

3   *Ibid.*

4   Suni, E., & Dimitriu, A., 'What is "revenge bedtime procrastination"?' www.sleepfoundation.org (2023) [accessed 25 April 2025].

5   Magalhães, P., *et al.*, 'An exploratory study on sleep procrastination: Bedtime vs. while-in-bed procrastination', *International Journal of Environmental Research and Public Health*, 17(16), 5892 (2020).

6   McRaven, W. H., *Make Your Bed* (Penguin, 2017).

7   Irwin, M. R., 'Sleep and inflammation: Partners in sickness and in health', *Nature Reviews Immunology*, 19(11) (2019), 702–715.

8   Cleveland Clinic, 'Insomnia', www.my.clevelandclinic.org [accessed 25 April 2025].

9   Seidler, A., et al., 'Seasonality of human sleep'.

10 Rizzolo, D., et al., 'Stress management strategies for students: The immediate effects of yoga, humor, and reading on stress', *Journal of College Teaching and Learning*, 6(8) (2009), 79–88.

11 Dawson, S. C., et al., 'Use of sleep aids in insomnia', *Primary Care Companion for CNS Disorders*, 25(3) (2023).

12 Hartwig, D., *The 4 Season Solution* (Thorsons HarperCollins, 2020).

Chapter 7: The fabric of winter

1   Lieber, J., & Bensmania, S., 'High-dimensional representation of texture in somatosensory cortex of primates', *Proceedings of the National Academy of Sciences*, 116(8) (2019), 3268–3277.

2   Wood, M., 'How the brain distinguishes textures—from sandpaper to silk', www.news.uchicago.edu (2019) [accessed 25 April 2025].

3   *Ibid.*

4   Antalis, 'What your hands make you remember – A study on the influence of touch and textures', www.antalis.co.uk (29 July 2020) [accessed 25 April 2025].

5 Spence, C., 'Shitsukan: The multisensory perception of quality', *Multisensory Research*, 33 (2020), 737–775.

6 Antalis, 'What your hands make you remember'.

7 Spence, C., 'Shitsukan'.

8 Etzi, R., Spence, C., & Gallace, A., 'Textures that we like to touch: An experimental study of aesthetic preferences for tactile stimuli', *Consciousness and Cognition*, 29 (2014), 178–188.

9 Racat, M., & Capelli, S., *Haptic Sensation and Consumer Behaviour: The Influence of Tactile Stimulation in Physical and Online Environments* (Palgrave Macmillan, 2020).

10 Etzi, R., Spence, C., & Gallace, A., 'Textures that we like to touch'.

11 Iosifyan, M., & Korolkova, O., 'Emotions associated with different textures during touch', *Consciousness and Cognition*, 71 (2019), 79–85.

12 Wainwright, A., *A Coast to Coast Walk* (Westmorland Gazette, 1973)

13 *The Verywell Mind Podcast with Amy Morin*, 'Episode 235 – Friday Fix: Surprising Ways Colors Affect How You Feel and Behave' (3 February 2023).

14 Jonauskaite, D., *et al.*, 'Universal patterns in color-emotion associations are further shaped by linguistic and geographic proximity', *Psychological Science*, 31(10) (2020), 1245–1260.

15 North American Mental Health Professional Advice Council (NAMHPAC), '7 Sad Colors at Home That Affect Your Mental State', www.namhpac.org (14 February 2020).

16 *Ibid.*

17 Küller, R., *et al.*, 'The impact of light and colour on psychological mood: A cross-cultural study of indoor work environments', *Ergonomics*, 49(14) (2006), 1496–1507.

Chapter 8: The taste of winter

1 Sahakian, B. J., & Labuzetta, J. N., *Bad Moves* (OUP, 2013).

2 Dunbar, R. I. M., 'Breaking Bread: The functions of social eating', *Adaptive Human Behavior and Physiology*, 3 (2017), 198–211.

3 *Ibid.*

4 Smith, M., 'Britons are as likely to eat dinner on the sofa as they are at a dining table', www.yougov.co.uk (2024) [accessed 25 April 2025].

5 Robinson, E., *et al.*, 'Eating attentively: A systematic review and meta-analysis of the effect of food intake memory and awareness on eating', *American Journal of Clinical Nutrition*, 97(4) (2013), 728–742.

6 Weisberger, M., 'Why do you usually eat the same thing for breakfast?' *Live Science* (22 February 2022).

Chapter 9: Winter's light

1 Vedant J., 'Sunsets in winter – simply spectacular', www.youngzine.org (4 March 2022).

Chapter 10: Getting out in winter

1 Deakin, R., *Notes from Walnut Tree Farm* (Penguin, 2009).

2 Jones, P., *A Winter Dictionary* (Elliott & Thompson Ltd, 2024).

3 Yankouskaya, A., *et al.*, 'The effects of whole-body cold-water immersion on brain connectivity related to the affective state in adults using fMRI: A protocol of a pre-post experimental design', *Bio-Protocol Journal*, 13(17) (2023).

4 Huttenen, P., Kokko, L., & Ylijukuri, V., 'Winter swimming improves general wellbeing', *International Journal of Circumpolar Health*, 63(2) (2004), 140–144.

5 Lindeman, S., Hirvonen, J., & Joukamaa, M., 'Neurotic psychopathology and alexithymia among winter swimmers and controls—a prospective study', *International Journal of Circumpolar Health*, 61(2) (2002), 123–130.

6 Hirvonen, J., *et al.*, 'Plasma catecholamines, serotonin and their metabolites and beta-endorphin of winter swimmers during one winter. Possible correlations to psychological traits', *International Journal of Circumpolar Health*, 61(4) (2002), 363–372.

Chapter 11: Moving through winter

1. Sports Insight, '61% Brits [sic] stop exercising completely during the winter months – new research reveals' (4 November 2022).

2. *Ibid.*

3. *Ibid.*

4. *Ibid.*

5. Peiser, B., 'Seasonal affective disorder and exercise treatment: A review', *Biological Rhythm Research*, 40(1) (2008), 85–97.

6. Burkeman, O., *Four Thousand Weeks* (Penguin, 2021).

7. '61% [sic] Brits stop exercising completely during the winter months'.

Chapter 12: Learning to love and celebrate in winter

1. Fitzgerald, S., 'Find light in the dark', *Psychologies* (February 2024).

Chapter 13: A calm(er) Christmas

1. Sherwood, H., 'Why is the Christian population of England and Wales declining?', *Guardian* (29 November 2022).

2. Smith, M., 'What kind of person doesn't like Christmas?', www.yougov.co.uk (18 December 2019) [accessed 25 April 2025].

3   Step Change Debt Charity, 'More than one in four people will struggle to afford Christmas this year, with around 4 million relying on credit', www.stepchange.org (11 December 2024) [accessed 25 April 2025].

4   www.warmwelcome.uk [accessed 25 April 2025].

Chapter 14: A winter garden

1   'The physiological effects of *Shinrin-yoku* (taking in the forest atmosphere or forest bathing): Evidence from field experiments in 24 forests across Japan', *US National Library of Medicine* (2 May 2009).

2   Waliczek, T. M., Bradley, J. C., & Zajicek, J. M., 'The effect of school gardens on children's interpersonal relationships and attitudes toward school', *HortTechnology*, 11(3) (2001), 466–468.

3   Ohly, H., *et al.*, 'A systematic review of the health and well-being impacts of school gardening: Synthesis of quantitative and qualitative evidence', *BMC Public Health*, 16(286) (2016).

4   Shanmuganathan-Felton, V., *et al.*, 'Cultivating wellbeing and mental health through gardening', www.bps.org.uk/psychologist (2020) [accessed 25 April 2025].

5   Barton, J., & Pretty, J., 'What is the best dose of nature and green exercise for improving mental health? A multi-study

analysis', *Environmental Science and Technology*, 44 (2010), 3947–3955.

6   Thompson, R., 'Gardening for health: A regular dose of gardening', *Clinical Medicine*, 18(3) (2018), 201–205.

7   'Gardening tips for winter', www.nationaltrust.org.uk [accessed 25 April 2025].

8   Walton Upchurch, M., 'Beauty in the winter garden: From the world's greatest gardens to your own private retreat, a well-designed garden will delight in winter', *Flower* (2021).

9   Aristotle (attrib.).

Chapter 15: The practical preparations for winter

1   Richter, M. *et al.*, 'Do words hurt? Brain activation during the processing of pain-related words', *Pain – The Journal for the International Association for the Study of Pain*, 148(2) (2010), 198–205.

2   de Bloom, J., Geurts, S. A. E., & Kompier, M. A. J., 'Vacation (after-) effects on employee health and well-being, and the role of vacation activities, experiences and sleep', *Journal of Happiness Studies*, 14 (2013), 613–633.

3   American Heart Association News, 'Are you drinking enough water during winter months?', www.heart.org (19 December 2019) [accessed 25 April 2025].

Chapter 16: A beginning, a middle and an end

1. Clear, J., *Atomic Habits* (Penguin, 2018).

Epilogue: The words of winter

1. Dent, S., *The Roots of Happiness* (Penguin, 2023).
2. Jones, P. A., *A Winter Dictionary* (Elliott & Thompson Ltd, 2024).

Index

alarms, setting 7, 24–5, 70–1
alcohol 227–8, 231–3, 236
ambiverts 172
amygdala 150–1
anxiety 22, 112, 140, 161, 199–200, 205
apricity 145, 146
Aristotle 213
Arnall, Cliff 30
art galleries 148
Atomic Habits 236
autumn 11–12, 27, 68–9, 77, 83, 137–8
avoidance 33

baking 63, 116, 118–23, 147, 165, 200
Baron, Naomi 91
beaches 57, 233
beauty of winter 84, 125, 128, 137–8, 142, 211, 221, 242
bedding, clean 81–2
bedrooms 79, 81–2, 84
bedtime 24, 68, 72–3, 199–200
being 86, 202, 239–40
bereavement 22–3
birds 203–4, 219
blankets 59, 61, 148, 223

blood pressure 81, 161, 204
blood sugar 159
Blue Monday 30–1, 219
body, repairing 15, 75
boundaries 35, 56, 194
bread, Grannie-Jo's 118–20
breakfast 109
breastfeeding 63
'broken record' technique 189
brooding 216–17
bulbs (garden) 208
bullying 187
Burkeman, Oliver 154

calendars
    empty 164–7
    re-writing 11–14, 36, 72
calmness 63, 86, 200–1, 214–15, 232
carbohydrates 21
celebrations 164
    Christmas 30, 48, 178–201
    negotiating with others 187–9
    of ourselves 170–5
    of winter 175–7
    see also festive season
cemeteries 220

charity 195–6
charity shops 95
chicks 216–17
children 47, 95, 180, 182, 188, 205, 237
Chinese Lantern Festival 130
chionophobia 212
Christianity 130, 178–9
Christmas 32, 48, 130, 175, 178–201, 230
  alone 184–6
  cost of 193–4, 223
  decorations 179
  emotions 197–9
  exhaustion from 189
  expectations of 183–8
  indulgence during 110
  long build-up to 9–11
  presents 179
  pressure and stress 180, 182
  reshaping 183–8, 200–1
  shopping 179–80, 218
  social significance 179
  staying calm 200–1
  supporting others 195–7
cities 220
  urban gardens 205
  in winter 135–7, 147–8
Clare, Horatio 3
cleaning 56, 131
Clear, James 236
clothes 232
  coats 94–5, 98–9
  dressing for the weather 92–4
  wardrobe audit 102–3
  for winter 59, 89–103, 223
colds 39–40, 75
cold-water immersion 143–4
colour 126, 202
  influence on mood 96–9
comedy gigs 166
comfort 5, 20, 42, 67, 89, 92, 158
comfort eating 106, 110–13
communication 98, 186–9, 194
community, connecting with 195–7, 249–50
commuting 140
compassion 20, 244
concentration 21, 70, 97, 204, 228
confelicity 252
cooking 191
  baking 63
  creating a cosy retreat 123–4
  for others 105–7
  recipes 114–15, 118–23
  in summer 116
  in winter 116–17
cortisol 71, 77, 143, 204
cosmognosis 54
cosy corners 84–5
courage 36, 246
Covid pandemic 46, 140
creativity 47, 57
crowds 135, 148
curry 113–15

dancing 56, 157, 163, 233, 250
darkness 125
  dangers of 155–6

daylight
    arranging work around 86–7
    duration 7, 69, 242
    and sleep 76–7
Deakin, Roger 138
decision fatigue 105–6
dehydration 228
depression 20, 31, 33, 97, 112, 140, 161, 167, 195, 205, 227, 326
    seasonal affective disorder (SAD) 2, 19–29, 46, 68, 69, 110, 140–2, 153, 167, 227
Die Hard 198
divorce 182
Diwali 130
dogs 60–1, 85, 252
    walking 137–43, 182
donating 195–7
dopamine 143, 195
drinks
    alcoholic 227–8, 231–2
    hot 86, 113, 228
    hydration 228
driving 6
droit a l'oubli 183, 201
Dún Laoghaire 143

emotions 16–17, 50, 217, 221
    at Christmas 197–9
endorphins 15, 29, 143
energy 17–18, 46, 245
    auditing 60–1
    'fall fatigue' 68
    and need for support 190–1

restoring 239, 241
small energy moments 131–2
timeline 17–18
equinoxes 11, 128
European Union 183
exercise 6–7, 15–16, 28, 150–63, 236
    different types 157–60
    in a group 157
    running 15–16, 157, 159–60, 236
    strength training 157–9
    yoga 54–5, 160–1, 232–3, 238
extroverts 172

fabrics 89
family 63, 180–2, 188, 192, 250, 253
fàng xīn 251
feefling 214
festive season
    build-up to 9–11
    celebrations 164–77
    Christmas 30, 48, 130, 175, 178–201
    indulgence during 110
    winter festivals 129–31, 176
films 198–9
finances 167, 193–4, 197
    planning ahead 222–4
fire 253
flowers 203, 208, 235
flu 75
food 21, 28, 57
    comfort eating 110–11
    eating with others 106, 108, 193

food – *cont'd.*
    and emotions 107
    food banks 196
    as medicine 112–13
    and memory 117–18
    root vegetables 104–5, 108–9
    seasonal 108–11
    unhealthy 226–7
    for winter 104–24
forest bathing 204
foxing days 149
friction, removing 218–19
friendship 249–50
    celebrating 169
frost 99, 138, 146, 148, 217

Galentine's Day 169
gardens and gardening 202–15
    impact on mental health 204–6
    as metaphors 206–12
    tidying and pruning 206–7
    winter beauty 210–11, 213
garlic 113
gemütlichkeit 250
genkan 218
gezelligheid 250
gifts 179, 192–3
ginger 112
gingerbread biscuits 121–3
glamour 99–100
gluggaveður 213
goals, setting 13, 32, 74, 226, 234–6, 238, 240
golden milk 113

grandparents 180–1
gratitude 241
grief 22–3
gym 6–7

Hanukkah 130
Hartwig, Dallas 87
health 39–40
    taking care of 226–8
heating 6, 158, 173, 212, 228
hibernacles 54, 249
hibernation 69, 132
HIIT (high intensity interval training) 154, 160
hippos 38–9, 41
hobbies, losing interest in 20
holidays 44–7, 52–3
    at home 56–8
home energy audit 60–1
hormones 15, 22, 77, 107, 218
houseplants 205–6
hydration 228
hygge 61–7, 116, 123, 223

ice 6, 139, 148
Iceland 145
illness 39–40
immune system 75
impulse control 218
industrialization 88
inflammation 112
insomnia 76, 82–4
introverts 172
isolation 168

journalling 35, 46, 222, 229

Kwanzaa 129–30

lagom 249
laptops 79, 80–1
letters, to future self 243–6
libraries 147, 214
lifestyle, seasonal adjustments 6–17
light
   beginning of lighter days 134
   daylight 7, 69, 76
   festivals celebrating 129–31
   light therapy 24–5, 28, 153
   and sleep 80
   in winter 125–34
The Light in the Dark 3
London 135, 220
loneliness 168, 181–2
love 168, 244
   of ourselves 169–75, 253
Lunar New Year 130, 165–7

manifestation 243
McRaven, William H. 73
melatonin 76–7, 81
memory 90, 107, 117–18, 204, 218
mental health 19–29, 140–4, 161
   and outdoor spaces 205–6
   taking care of 226–8
   see also depression; seasonal affective disorder (SAD)
meteorological seasons 11–12

mindsets, shifting 51, 219–20
minimalism 96
money 167, 193–4, 197
   savings 222–4
mood 30, 50, 168
   see also seasonal affective disorder (SAD)
moon 87
morning people 16
motivation 48, 97, 101, 150, 154, 156, 160, 239
museums 148

nature 6, 146
   as cyclical 210, 235
   engaging with 204–15
negativity 221–2
nest-building 219
New Year 30–1, 170
   adjusting 12–14, 229
   Lunar 130, 165–7
   resolutions 72, 158, 234–7
   ways of celebrating 231–4
night, being awake during 82–6
novelty 154–5

ohana 249–50
outdoors 137–9
   gardens 202–15
Oxford 135–6
oxytocin 15, 29

pain 112
Palentine's Day 169

parenthood 63, 64, 180, 182
parks 135, 155, 204–5
parties 110–11
peiskos 253
phones 79, 80, 152
　scrolling before bed 75
photography 211
planning 42, 47, 216–28, 229, 235–7
plants 202–3
　growing 205–7
pollution 70, 126
preparations
　for end of winter 203, 229, 241–2
　for winter 28, 77, 95, 101, 167, 216–28, 243
presents 179, 181, 191–3
prinkling 195, 248–9
productivity 51–2, 55, 206
protein 109–10
rain 3, 13, 93, 137, 146
Rayleigh scattering 125
reading 56, 61, 80–1, 90–1
reassurance 204, 251
recipes
　Grannie-Jo's bread 118–20
　Super Healing Curry 114–15
　ultimate gingerbread biscuits 121–3
reflection 33–8, 56, 230, 243–4
relaxation 40, 46, 56, 58–9, 65, 79, 140, 227, 233, 249, 251
religion 10, 129, 178–9

resetting 31, 52
resting 3, 6, 40, 46, 71, 74–5, 111, 161, 249
retreats 129, 225, 249
　at home 54–67, 85, 123–4, 172, 176, 249
revenge bedtime procrastination (RBP) 72–3, 94
Richard, Cliff 44
right to be forgotten 183, 201
rituals 55, 80, 176–7
roast dinners 105
roses 207–8
routines 6–8, 226
　adjusting 15–16, 71
running 15–16, 157, 159–60, 236

safety 155–6, 251
savings 223
school holidays 47, 53, 154
screen brightness 80–1
seasonal adjustments 5–18, 68–9
　creating seasonal spaces 58–61
seasonal affective disorder (SAD) 2, 19–29, 46, 68, 69, 110, 140–2, 153, 167, 227
seasons, defining 11–12
secret Santa 194
security 251
sedentary lifestyle 153, 157
self-acceptance 170–5, 234–5, 253
sensory memories 90
serotonin 21, 143
sex 79, 80

sheets, clean 81–2
shinrin-yoku 204
shitsukan 91
shoes 218–19
shopping 179–80, 218, 225–6
sleep 28, 64, 68–88
   hygiene 77–8
   hypersomnia 21
   insomnia 76, 82–4
   as recharging 74
   schedules 78
   seasonal changes in 68–71, 78
   types of 70
sleepovers 233
slowing down 8, 32, 240, 245, 248
snow 139, 212–15
   words for 214
social events 32, 50, 147, 164–77, 222
social media 75, 78, 152, 198, 221
softness 59, 89–92, 100, 232, 248
soil 209
solstice 31–2, 175, 229
soups 108
spices 112–13, 116
spirituality 129–30
spontaneity 166
spring 11–13, 74, 134
   flowers 208
   preparing for 161, 203, 208, 241–2
stews 105, 108
stimulation 6, 153
strength training 157–9
stress 152, 205–6

suicide 21
summer 8, 12–14, 104, 129, 136, 154–5, 250
   clothes 93–4, 96, 100
   food 5, 116
   holidays 44–5, 47
sunrise 125–8, 156, 221, 233
   lamps 24–5, 81
sunset 24, 80, 126–8
Super Healing Curry 114–15
support
   needing 190–1, 244–6
   networks 156–7
   supporting others 195–7
surprises 192–3
swimming, open-water 143–5
systems, setting up 238–9

tasks, and goals 238
tax year 12, 14
tea 6–7, 61, 112, 121, 203
temperature 46, 85, 93, 95, 143, 150, 157, 196, 213
textures 89–92, 97
Thailand 45
tidying 66, 133
TikTok 152
time wasting 40, 230
to-do lists 42, 203
tourism 135–6
traditions 180–2
   changing and forgetting 183–4
trauma 161
trees 13, 34, 204–5, 210

Tripadvisor 44
trygghet 251
turmeric 112–13
TV 61, 78, 80–1
Upchurch, Mary Walton 210–11

Valentine's Day 168–9
vitamin D 46, 153
   supplements 26–8
vocabulary 247–53
volunteering 195–6

Wainwright, Alfred 92
walking 56, 137–43, 146–8, 152, 156, 182, 248
wallowing 38–43
wardrobe audit 102–3
Warm Welcome Space 196
warmth 85, 212–13, 253
wasting time 40, 230
water 7, 228
weather 92–3, 126–7, 137, 146–7
   snow 212–15
weight gain 110
wildlife 139, 203, 210
winding down 48–9, 224–5
winter
   beauty of 210–11, 213, 217, 221
   beginning 228, 230–8
   blues 33, 227; *see also* seasonal affective disorder (SAD)
   breaks 44–7, 52–3
   defining 11–12
   end 228, 241–2
   making adjustments for 5–18
   middle 228, 230, 239–40
   retreats 54–67
   vocabulary 247–53
woodlands 204–5
work
   pressures of 48–51, 224–5
   workloads 51–2
worry time 199–200

yoga 54–5, 160–1, 232–3, 238
yutori 248

Notes